D0114496

TALES FROM THE MORGUE

FORENSIC ANSWERS
TO NINE
FAMOUS CASES

INCLUDING THE
SCOTT PETERSON &
CHANDRA LEVY CASES

TALES FROM THE MORGUE

CYRIL WECHT, MD, JD
and MARK CURRIDEN
with ANGELA POWELL

Palisades Park Public Library
257 Second Street
Palisades Park, NJ 07650

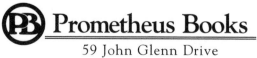 Prometheus Books
59 John Glenn Drive
Amherst, New York 14228-2197

Published 2005 by Prometheus Books

Tales from the Morgue: Forensic Answers to Nine Famous Cases. Copyright © 2005 by Cyril Wecht, Mark Curriden, and Angela Powell. All rights reserved. No part of this publication may be reproduced, stored in a retrieval system, or transmitted in any form or by any means, digital, electronic, mechanical, photocopying, recording, or otherwise, or conveyed via the Internet or a Web site without prior written permission of the publisher, except in the case of brief quotations embodied in critical articles and reviews.

Inquiries should be addressed to
Prometheus Books
59 John Glenn Drive
Amherst, New York 14228–2197
VOICE: 716–691–0133, ext. 207
FAX: 716–564–2711
WWW.PROMETHEUSBOOKS.COM

09 08 07 06 05   5 4 3 2 1

Library of Congress Cataloging-in-Publication Data

Wecht, Cyril H., 1931–
    Tales from the morgue : forensic answers to nine famous cases / Cyril Wecht and Mark Curriden with Angela Powell ; foreword by Robert K. Tanenbaum.
        p. cm.
    Includes bibliographical references and index.
    ISBN 1–59102–353–X (hardcover : alk. paper)
    1. Forensic pathology—Case studies. 2. Death—Causes—Case studies. 3. Criminal investigation—Case studies. I. Curriden, Mark. II. Powell, Angela. III. Title.

RA1063.4.W437 2005
614'.1—dc22

                                                              2005017805

Printed in the United States of America on acid-free paper

614.1
WEC

Wecht, Cyril H.,
Tales from the morgue :forensic answers
Prometheus Books,2005.
39153090412976
Palisades Park Library

For my dear wife Sigrid

CHW

For our daughter Darby—thank you for being such a fabulous kid

MC and AP

CONTENTS

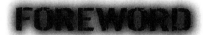

FOREWORD

ROBERT K. TANENBAUM

Greatness is more than achieving proficiency in one's craft. The true champion is one who elevates his profession through excellence that is derived from a courageous heart and a pure soul. The individual who so triumphs evinces a passion and energy that inspires others. In public life, a heroic figure enhances the dignity of his office during his tenure by serving the ends of justice. He respects our laws and values, and serves passionately the truth. He takes no shortcuts, seeks no loopholes, and possesses a soul that is nonnegotiable. Dr. Cyril Wecht is America's foremost distinguished medical examiner. More than sitting atop the "greasy pole" of his profession, Dr. Cyril Wecht is a great man. He has in painstaking fashion committed himself to seeking truth. He possesses the heart and courage of the warrior. His opinions are honestly derived from the documented evidence.

Dr. Wecht brings a unique commitment to our justice system. He understands the crucial role he plays in it. The medical examiner is an essential participant in the justice system's search for truth. The medical examiner must be independent. His opinion ought never be compromised to satisfy a prosecution theory. The

9

medical examiner is on no one's team. He is a scientist who during the course of a murder case opines as to cause and manner of death.

Tales from the Morgue is much more than superb reportage about fascinating and mysterious murder cases. Its essence lies in understanding the motivation and passion of Dr. Cyril Wecht. He rages against injustice. He anguishes for those who are unjustly accused. He is unwilling to permit corrupt justice system officials to railroad innocent people on false or inadequate evidence.

After reading this book, I am convinced that Dr. Wecht could have readily authored President Lincoln's words: "I pity the man who cannot feel the pain of the lash placed upon another." For how nightmarish it must be to be unjustly convicted and incarcerated. Each case documented in *Tales from the Morgue* cries out for compassion, understanding, and justice.

No legitimate commentary of this book can be given without noting the important contribution of Dr. Wecht's collaborator, Mark Curriden. Mr. Curriden, in his own right, is a brilliant author and also a crusader for justice.

Robert K. Tanenbaum
Attorney at Law

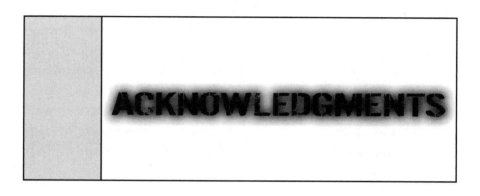

ACKNOWLEDGMENTS

There are several key people we would like to personally thank for helping us with the research, writing, and editing of this book.

Dr. Henry Lee, Dr. Michael Baden, and Dr. Tom Noguchi are good friends and colleagues. But they also provided us their invaluable insights and experiences in the cases in which Dr. Wecht was involved with them. Without their assistance and guidance, this book would not have been possible.

There are no two people who are more knowledgeable of the facts and evidence in the assassination of President John F. Kennedy than Dr. Gary Aguilar and Robert Groden. We thank them for their help.

The Digman and Gammage families deserve our thanks and our admiration for seeking the truth in their respective cases. They have faced tragedy, and yet they have stood strong. We owe them a debt of gratitude.

The investigative reporting skills of television journalist Terri Taylor must be mentioned. Without her, the story of what happened in Gander, Newfoundland, might never have been uncov-

11

ered. In addition, the *Modesto Bee* and Court TV need to be praised for their voluminous and exceptional coverage in the Jayson Williams and Scott Peterson trials.

The world of the Internet was also helpful. There are a myriad of Web sites about Marilyn Monroe, but we found Danamo's Marilyn Monroe Online at http://marilynmonroepages.com/ and Marilyn Monroe's official Web site, http://www.marilynmonroe.com/, to be accurate sources of information. The History Channel's Web site and www.historymatters.com were tremendously helpful.

We would be remiss if we did not thank the folks at Prometheus Books, particularly our editor, Linda Regan. She did her best to keep us grammatically correct and on a time schedule. Thanks must also go out to Jason Curriden, who helped edit before the edits, and to our families, who put up with us.

Finally, a personal expression of gratitude goes to Kathy McCabe and Flo Johnson, who daily help keep Dr. Wecht operating efficiently and professionally.

INTRODUCTION

The current intense interest in forensic science has been fueled by the success of recent TV shows such as *Crossing Jordan* and *Forensic Files*. Sherlock Holmes, Hercule Poirot, and Charlie Chan have given way to *CSI* and *Quincy*. The murder cases and controversial deaths depicted in *Tales from the Morgue* will take you beyond fiction, into the real-life world of the forensic pathologist examining the body at the death scene and into the morgue in an effort to recognize, collect, and analyze all that may ultimately lead to the conviction of the assailant or the exoneration of the innocent.

The fictional dramatization of highly skilled forensic scientists solving complex murder cases and other major crimes may have been an important factor in stimulating the public's fascination with forensic scientific investigation and the popularity this field currently enjoys throughout much of the world. However, the occurrence of highly controversial, notorious, and well-publicized real-life cases such as the Laci and Connor Peterson murder, the Chandra Levy homicide, John F. Kennedy's assassination, the death of Marilyn Monroe, the inexplicable deadly crash of a military plane transporting hundreds of soldiers, and many others has

13

made millions of people aware of the significant and essential role that forensic pathologists and other forensic scientists play in criminal investigations. Actual trials are often reported in great detail by broadcast and print news media. Indeed, some cases are covered live and even acquire an audience that rivals the most popular network television programs.

The investigation of violent, sudden, suspicious, unexpected, unexplained, and medically unattended deaths in order to determine the cause, mechanism, and manner of death is the primary responsibility of the forensic pathologist. Quite often it is also necessary to ascertain the time and place of death; the relationship between natural disease and death; and when two or more victims are found at the same location, the sequence of their deaths.

Welcome to the world of forensic pathology, where mystery meets science, law and medicine join forces, and amazing discoveries lurk around every corner. Most important, it is a world where the application of fundamental scientific principles and sound investigative techniques can help to uncover the truth and ensure that justice is served. Mention the term *forensic pathologist* and most people think of *Quincy* and fictional *CSI* television heroes. Unlike a typical plot from the TV series, however, not every murder or medical intrigue is solved in sixty minutes by looking through a microscope or by examining the soles of a dead man's feet, as Jack Klugman's character was apt to do.

This book was written to take you inside some of the nation's most bizarre and intriguing medicolegal investigations and show you how forensic scientists help to solve crimes—and likewise how they sometimes fail to solve them.

Technically defined, forensic pathology is that field of medicine that is concerned with the investigation of sudden, violent, suspicious, unexpected, unexplained, or medically unattended deaths.

The most widely used courtroom expert in criminal cases is the forensic pathologist. Why? Quite simply because there is no other medical specialist as critically integrated into the legal process. In theory, it has always been this way. But it was not until fairly recently that the usefulness of the forensic pathologist was fully appreciated.

As I look back over my nearly forty-five-year career as a forensic pathologist, I am repeatedly reminded of the old French adage "The more things change, the more they remain the same." For all of the advances I have witnessed in my field over the past four decades, the discipline's fundamental concepts have not changed all that much. Even today, a shooting is still a shooting, a stabbing is still a stabbing, and a beating is still a beating. Every year people die in plane crashes, in fires, in bombings, in falls. And it remains my job to determine just how these deaths occurred. It may sound like a horror story, but that's what forensic pathology is all about, and that's what it always will be about.

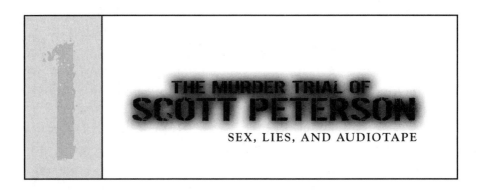

1

SEX, LIES, AND AUDIOTAPE

s murder trials go, *The People v. Scott Peterson* had it all. The victims were a young, vivacious, pregnant substitute school teacher and her unborn son. The defendant was a handsome, philandering fertilizer salesman. The alleged motive was sex and money, lies and betrayal. The "cast" also included an attractive mistress-turned-embittered undercover informant, a high-profile lawyer, feuding families, and national media attention.

And, of course, it took place in California, where six-day trials last four months and where no one can ever predict what the jury will do.

I was hired in the summer of 2003 by Scott Peterson's lawyer, Mark Geragos, to examine the forensic and scientific evidence in the deaths of Laci and Conner Peterson. I performed a second autopsy on the pair. I also visited the alleged crime scene, as well as the locations where the victims' bodies were found. In addition, I reviewed the state's entire case against Scott Peterson.

But let me not get ahead of myself.

The story of Scott and Laci Peterson officially began at 10:18 AM on December 24, 2002. That is when Karen Servas, their neighbor, arrived home after some early morning Christmas shopping. She had just purchased some holiday ornaments to decorate her house. As she started to enter her home, she noticed the neighbor's dog, a golden retriever named McKenzie, wandering around outside with his leash in tow. "The leash had—it was dirty; it had leaves and grass clippings on it," she said. "It was moist."[1]

Mrs. Servas grabbed the dog's leash to take him back to his home. She noted that her neighbors' front gate was closed and locked, but their side gate was partially open. Since she saw no one inside, she led the retriever into the neighbors' backyard and returned to her home.

Late that afternoon, Scott Peterson returned home after trying out his new fishing boat in the San Francisco Bay. Laci, his twenty-seven-year-old wife, was nowhere to be seen. Scott and Laci, who was eight months pregnant with their first child, had been married for five years.

Scott immediately removed his clothes and threw them in the couple's washing machine. In the backyard, he spotted McKenzie. His leash was still attached. Laci's car, a Land Rover, was still in the driveway.

A few minutes later, he picked up the telephone. His first call was to one of his best friends, a neighbor named Greg Reed. "Have you or Kristen talked to Laci today or yesterday?" Scott asked in a voice mail that Reed described as frantic.[2]

Next he called Laci's parents. He told Laci's stepfather, Ron Grantski, that he had just returned from a day of golfing and that Laci wasn't home. Had she been at their house or called them? Scott inquired.

Neither of Laci's parents had seen or heard from their daughter. Laci's stepfather immediately feared something bad had happened and called the Modesto Police Department.

Over the next few hours, police joined family and friends gathering at the Petersons' home. Family members comforted one another, praying that Laci was safe or had decided to go shopping with a friend. Every time the door opened, all heads would turn, hoping it would be Laci.

A handful of police officers spoke with each member of the family, garnering as much information about Laci as possible in order to organize a successful search. They obtained recent photographs to distribute electronically throughout the state. The first person they questioned, of course, was Scott. After all, he was the last person to see her alive and the person who knew her best.

What was she doing when he left to go fishing?

What was she wearing?

Had she been upset?

Did she say if she had any plans to meet with friends or go shopping?

Scott told the officers that when he had left that morning at 9:30 AM, his wife was wearing black stretch pants and jewelry that she had inherited from her grandmother. He said that she had been mopping the kitchen floor while watching *Martha Stewart Living* and had planned to take McKenzie for a walk through East La Loma Park, which was not far from their home. The initial concern was that Laci had fallen down, hurt herself, and was either lying unconscious or in dire need of medical help.

For several hours that evening and into the night, officers, family, friends, and neighbors searched the park and their local community for Laci. They worked the telephones, calling everyone they could think of, to ask if they had seen Laci. Every hospital and doctor's office was checked. No one slept that Christmas Eve.

There were only a handful of possibilities: Laci had injured herself and was unable to notify her family; she had fled and did not want anyone to know where she was; she had been kidnapped; or she was the victim of a violent crime. Scott's and Laci's families immediately dismissed the idea that Laci would leave voluntarily for such a long period of time without letting one of them know.

Scott and other family members started their Christmas morning at the break of dawn by organizing another search throughout their neighborhood and the nearby park. Janet Kenworthy, who lived in the same neighborhood as the Petersons, was walking her white husky named Aroo in the park when she bumped into Scott. "He reached into his coat, pulls out a flyer and says, 'My wife is missing,'" according to Kenworthy. "He about broke down in front of me. I did see tears, retain-your-composure efforts. I would have sworn at that time that he was innocent."[3]

By late morning, the Modesto police were starting to believe that Laci Peterson was probably the victim of foul play. The department brought in its detective division to investigate. The Petersons' home was "neat, clean and organized," according to initial police reports.[4] Det. Al Brocchini was the first to officially question Scott Peterson, and he didn't mince words:

"You guys haven't had any marriage problems?" Brocchini asked.

"No," Peterson responded.

"Everything is good," the detective asked again.

"Yes," Peterson said again.[5]

Later that afternoon, Modesto police detective Craig Grogan interviewed Scott for three hours. Scott told the investigator that Laci seemed happy and upbeat when he left to go fishing. Detective Grogan reported that Scott was very cooperative, even suggesting that it was possible that a homeless vagrant may have attacked her as she walked the dog through the park, in order to steal Laci's jewelry. In searching the house, police found that Laci's tennis shoes, a pair of diamond earrings, and a diamond-encrusted Croton watch were missing.[6]

Scott told the detective that he left his house at about 9:30 AM to go fishing by himself in his new fourteen-foot aluminum boat. He said he had put his boat in the water at the Berkeley Marina and had motored to a spot off Brooks Island. He provided the authorities with a ticket stub showing that he had parked at the marina and how long he had been there. Scott also admitted that he had washed his clothes immediately after returning home from his fishing trip because they had gotten wet from "fishing and raining"—something that seemed suspicious to the detectives.[7]

As Christmas Day wore on, more and more law enforcement officers joined the case. Douglas Mansfield, an investigator and chief polygraph expert with the California Department of Justice, asked Scott if he would be willing to take a lie-detector test. Scott declined, saying that he was emotionally and psychologically upset about his wife's disappearance and that he had heard polygraph examinations were unreliable. But Scott did reiterate that he and Laci were a happy family and had been faithful to each other.

"There are no third parties," Scott told Mansfield.[8]

On December 26 the search for Laci expanded to neighborhoods beyond where the Petersons lived. Thousands of fliers featuring Laci's photograph were distributed throughout Modesto and beyond. Laci's family, with Scott in the background, went on national television to plead for their daughter's safe return. They announced that a reward fund had been created for anyone who had information regarding Laci's whereabouts. Their reward would eventually grow to more than $500,000.

The next day, detectives obtained warrants from a local judge to search the Petersons' home and Scott's warehouse. Detectives called in their forensic experts to scour Scott and Laci's house. The officers found the warehouse where Scott operated his fertilizer business to be "a mess" and "very disorganized." On the floor, they found five "voided circular" patches. Scott told the authorities that he had used the cement to build an eight-pound anchor for his new boat, which had left the circular patterns. However, the detective wondered if the cement had been used as weights to sink Laci's body.[9]

The police officers asked Scott if he would strip to his boxers so they could examine his body for possible scratches or other signs of an altercation. Scott consented, but the officers found nothing.

Even so, the police declined to identify Scott Peterson as a suspect. Nor did they rule him out.

That being said, it was logical for the police to include Scott as a suspect. As Detective Grogan later admitted, Scott became a textbook suspect "based on the fact that he is close to the victim, the fact that he was the last person to see her, the fact that he discovered her missing, the fact that she disappeared when he was by himself on what appeared to be an unusual trip for him, not part of his normal behavior."[10]

Based on my experience, including four decades of homicide investigations, it certainly made sense for the police to consider Scott a suspect from day one. Husbands, wives, boyfriends, and girlfriends are always going to be suspects, at least initially. Police start a homicide investigation by focusing first on the immediate family, and then neighbors, coworkers, and business associates.

On New Year's Eve, nearly one thousand friends, family, and supporters gathered at a candlelight service in the park. They prayed, sang hymns, and shared their memories and thoughts of the missing woman.

Laci Denise Rocha was born in Modesto on May 4, 1975. She was raised on a California dairy farm and had been a cheerleader in high school. Her stepfather referred to her as "jabber-jaws" because she talked so much as a child. Laci attended college at California Polytechnic State University.

Scott, who was born in San Diego in 1972, also was a student at Cal Poly at the time he met Laci. He was working at the Pacific Café, which Laci frequented. Laci thought Scott was cute and had a friend give him her phone number. It didn't take him long to call.

Three years older than Laci, Scott was an outdoorsman who loved sports, fishing, and hunting. He also had a passion for golf and had been high school classmates with professional golfer Phil Mickelson.

Starting on January 4, 2003, and lasting for several days, professional divers searched the San Francisco Bay and the area around the Berkeley Marina, where Scott had been fishing. They turned up nothing. Then, a week later, electronic sonar detected something large in the bay. Divers, believing it might be Laci's body, again spent a day underwater. But the object turned out to be an anchor.

As Laci's disappearance became a national news story, Scott faded further and further into the background. He seldom appeared or spoke at press conferences. He didn't seem overly emotional and was even caught on videotape laughing and joking while talking on his cell phone. This occurred during the candlelight vigil in East La Loma Park on New Year's Eve.

But when reporters asked Laci's family if they thought Scott was a suspect, Laci's mother, Sharon Rocha, didn't hesitate a second before dismissing the idea that her son-in-law had anything to do with her daughter's disappearance. On January 13, Scott's father, Lee Peterson, joined Sharon Rocha, Ron Grantski, and Laci's sister, Amy Rocha, for a live interview on CNN's *Larry King Live*.

Larry King: Sharon, from all you knew, is this a very happy marriage, the Peterson marriage?

Sharon Rocha: Yes. They just are really truly in love with each other. They do everything together. They're partners. They're a team. They love each other. They planned together, they play together. They're always smiling. They're just very happy, well-adjusted couple. Never been any indication, I never heard Laci say she was even angry with Scott for any reason at all.

Larry: So, therefore, Ron, there is no thought in your mind, obviously people always suspect the most immediate family member and the husband has not been released from that suspicion, but there was no question in your mind that he's not involved, right, Ron?

Ron Grantski: Well, that's correct. I, you know, it might seem unusual he went fishing by himself, but I go fishing by myself a lot. Heaven forbid something happened here because I do it all the time.

Larry: So that's not strange to you that he would go fishing?

Ron: No. Not to me.

Larry: Amy, as far as you knew, is your sister very happily married?

Amy Rocha: Very happily married, yes.

Larry: So you join your stepfather and your mother in saying that you don't question at all Scott's involvement?

Amy: We have no question in our mind about Scott; he's part of our family.

Larry: One of the things that does come up, Lee, why Scott doesn't appear for interviews. Do you know why?

Lee Peterson: Yes. Well, he's very emotional. He would—he would break down. He wouldn't be able to finish an interview. And he doesn't want the media focus on him, he wants it on having Laci's picture in front of the nation so that someone may report something and we can get her back in our family.[11]

The interview showed how Laci's family trusted their son-in-law. Three days later, Scott Peterson's relationship with his wife's family took a dramatic shift. On January 16 Modesto police, in a private meeting, informed Laci's parents that Scott had been having an affair with a twenty-seven-year-old masseuse. The detectives also told the family that Scott had taken out a $250,000 life insurance policy on Laci. From that point on, their relationship was never the same. Laci's family knew that Scott had betrayed their daughter—and had betrayed them.

On January 24 Modesto police called a press conference in which they introduced Amber Frey—the other woman. A tall, attractive, single mother from Fresno, Frey told reporters that she and Scott met on November 20, 2002. They had been on four dates. Throughout, Scott had told her he was not married. In fact, she said Scott had told her in mid-December that he had recently lost his wife and that this would be his first Christmas alone. Frey's press conference was carried live on CNN and received national news attention.

It didn't take long for Laci's family to respond. "I trusted him and

I stood by him in the initial phases of my sister's disappearance," Brent Rocha, Laci's brother, told reporters. "However, Scott has not been forthcoming with information regarding my sister's disappearance. I'm only left to question what else he may be hiding."[12]

Four days later, Scott appeared on ABC-TV's *Good Morning America* in a one-on-one interview with Diane Sawyer in the quietness of his own home and without a lawyer present. He cried when talking about his missing wife and their unborn son. He claimed he had nothing to do with Laci's disappearance, and he denied that he had killed her. Scott confessed to the affair, which he said he had told police about right away. He also said that he had told his wife about the affair and that, while Laci was angry about it, she had made peace with it. Finally, he told Diane that he and Laci had purchased $250,000 life insurance policies for each other the year before.[13]

As the investigation continued, police focused more and more on Scott. In February prosecutors informed Scott that if he would confess and help them find Laci's body, they would agree not to seek the death penalty against him. Peterson rejected the offer because he said he was innocent and did not know the whereabouts of Laci's body.[14]

Both sides of the family held vigils and daylong searches for Laci in late January, as the date she was expected to give birth approached. That week I was a guest on Greta Van Susteren's show, *On the Record*, on Fox News. Greta asked me if I believed that Laci was still alive.

"I would like to hope and pray that she is," I told Greta. "But I am not optimistic. It has been a month now since Laci disappeared. No one has heard from her. No one had seen her. Where would she go? Who would she stay with? Who would kidnap and keep an eight-month-pregnant woman without ransom? You have to look at what the likely scenarios are. Unfortunately, none of them legitimately point to Laci still being alive. I hope that I'm wrong."

On February 18 Modesto detectives descended on Scott

Peterson's house with a new search warrant. For ten hours, police combed through the home. They seized Scott's new truck and nearly one hundred personal items from the house. Two weeks later, authorities officially reclassified Laci Peterson from "missing person" to "homicide."

Between December 25 and the beginning of April, Modesto police reported receiving more than eight thousand tips from concerned citizens. One of the tipsters was Vivian Mitchell, a neighbor of Scott and Laci's. She left a voice mail message on the police tip line that she had seen Laci walking her dog sometime between 10 and 10:15 AM on December 24—about forty-five minutes after Scott Peterson left his house to go fishing. However, Mitchell said police never called her back.[15]

But the biggest tip came the morning of April 13. Michael Looby was walking his dog along the east shore of the San Francisco Bay when he noticed what appeared to be a baby's body lying in grassy marshland that was dotted with trash. A storm the evening before had washed debris all along the shoreline. The baby's body rested at the high-tide watermark, meaning it had probably only been there since the storm. The next day another dog walker, Elena Gonzalez, was chasing one of her dogs at a park in Point Isabel when she spotted what she first thought was a bloated seal carcass wedged in some rocks; it was partially submerged in water along the bay shoreline.[16]

On April 18 authorities confirmed that the bodies recovered in the San Francisco Bay were those of Laci and Conner Peterson.

Modesto police, who had been using electronic surveillance and other methods to track Scott's movements, spotted Scott that afternoon in his car near the Torrey Pines Golf Course in La Jolla, just south of San Diego. This was more than four hundred miles from his home in Modesto and not far from the Mexican border. The detectives, who were in unmarked police cars, pulled behind Scott's vehicle, a maroon Mercedes sedan, and hit their flashing blue lights. Scott immediately pulled over.

Det. Jon Buehler, who had been working on the Laci Peterson case from the start, asked Scott to step out of the car. When he did, the detective applied handcuffs and informed Peterson that he was under arrest for the murders of his wife and unborn son. Under California law, a fetus over the age of seven weeks can be considered a murder victim. By officially charging Scott with two murders, prosecutors were also allowed to seek the death penalty as punishment, according to state law.

Scott's hair and goatee were bleached blond. Detectives discovered an envelope in his car containing $14,932 in cash. He also had Mexican currency, his brother's driver's license, and credit cards in the names of his mother and half sister. Detective Buehler said Peterson's car was also stocked with survivalist equipment, including several changes of clothes, a water purifier, an axe, a saw, and three knives. Police and prosecutors contended that Scott was preparing to flee to Mexico to avoid being arrested.

That afternoon California attorney general Bill Lockyer called the case against Scott Peterson a "slam dunk case."[17] Prosecutors also announced they were seeking the death penalty.

When I heard the attorney general of California announce in a live press conference that their case against Scott Peterson was a slam dunk, I was impressed. I had no insider information about the case and had been following the investigation through the newspapers and cable television news programs. I knew only what the media had reported. But when the state's attorney general declared that they had a slam-dunk case, I figured that they had evidence the public didn't know about. Slam-dunk cases are those where the defendant has confessed. Slam-dunk cases usually mean there is a videotape of the crime, multiple eyewitnesses, or overwhelming physical evidence, such as DNA or fingerprints.

My official involvement in the Peterson case began in mid-summer, when criminal defense attorney Mark Geragos called me at my office to see if I was interested in conducting a second autopsy on Laci and Conner. Geragos and I had actually been guest commentators or analysts discussing the case on CNN, MSNBC, and on Greta Van Susteren's show. But that was prior to Geragos being hired to defend Scott Peterson by Peterson's family. I told Geragos during that initial phone call that I was pretty certain I could do it but that I needed a few days to make sure.

A few days later, I learned from my good friend and colleague Dr. Henry Lee that Geragos had also called him. Henry had agreed to join the defense team. Henry is the chief emeritus of the Connecticut State Forensic Science Laboratory, which handles all forensic examinations, such as DNA testing, for law enforcement in Connecticut. He also is a distinguished professor at the University of New Haven's Henry C. Lee Institute of Forensic Science. Henry and I have known each other for many years. We have been to each other's homes and been involved in scores of cases together, including the investigations into O. J. Simpson, Chandra Levy, and the JFK assassination.

With news that Henry had joined the defense team, I called Mark Geragos back a couple days later to let him know I was onboard.

"I look forward to examining all this evidence the prosecution and police have collected," I told Geragos.

"There's not much," he responded. "But we will send you what they've given to us."

A week later, Geragos sent to me via Federal Express a package that contained the state's official autopsy reports on Laci and Conner, the official police investigative report, and medical records from Laci's gynecologist. Geragos was right—there wasn't much to it. The autopsy reports were quite vague and nondescript with very few conclusions. In fact, I was surprised at the brevity of the report, which was a mere two pages long.

In a high-profile case like this, I thought that the medical examiner's report would have been much more detailed. Some medical examiners deliberately keep their autopsy reports short and do not go into any detailed conclusions or analysis. This allows them to adjust or modify their courtroom testimony without being held account-able for earlier, seemingly contradictory, findings. The investigative report was equally as general, providing very little insight into what physical or forensic evidence the state had collected.

The one thing that jumped out at me was on the Conner Peterson autopsy report. The medical examiner who performed the autopsy described the body as being that of a "full-term" baby. That was strange because Laci was only eight-months pregnant when she disappeared. Her due date wasn't until early February. If the body was that of Conner, as the DNA testing showed, and it was full-term, then there were only two possible conclusions: Laci was alive until at least the middle of January when she gave birth or the baby was removed from her and kept alive for a short period. Either way, this would be favorable news for Scott Peterson because it meant that one or both of them had been killed days or weeks after Scott was the focus of twenty-hour-a-day surveillance by the Modesto police. A third possibility was that the autopsy report was simply wrong.

In a series of telephone conferences during the next several days, Henry and I agreed that it would be best if we conducted our own examination of the bodies. The next week, Geragos filed a court motion, asking the judge to issue an order that required Stanislaus County prosecutors and Modesto police to allow us to conduct a second autopsy on the bodies of Laci and Conner.

Judge Alfred A. Delucchi agreed. Henry and I flew to San Francisco the second week of August. We were met at the airport by an investigator who worked for Geragos on the Peterson case. That evening we spent several hours at our hotel in a conference room, going over the evidence in the case with Geragos and his legal team. They had prepared a PowerPoint presentation that walked us through the timeline of the case—from the point when Scott went fishing and Laci became missing to the finding of the bodies in mid-April.

At 8:30 the next morning, August 12, Geragos drove us to the

Contra Costa County coroner's office. The bodies were being held by Contra Costa County officials instead of Stanislaus County because that was the official jurisdiction where the bodies were discovered. As we arrived at the sheriff's office, which is where the coroner performed his autopsies, we were met by a throng of television, radio, newspaper, and magazine reporters. Someone had tipped them off that we were coming. We waved politely, but declined to make any public comments.

The autopsy examination room was not large—the size of a small or medium-sized bedroom. It had one autopsy table in the middle. There were a couple of cabinets on the walls that contained protective gloves and other examination materials. There were five people present from the defense side—Geragos, another lawyer from his firm, the investigator, Henry, and myself. The Stanislaus County district attorney's office sent one of its prosecutors as well as a couple of detectives. Despite eight people crammed into such a small room, we had ample space in which to conduct our examination.

After we introduced ourselves, there was no friendly chatter. The milieu was very businesslike and professional.

The bodies were being held in the room next door in standard morgue coolers. The coolers are maintained between thirty-eight and forty degrees, which keeps bodies from decaying further. The key is to keep the bodies cold without freezing them. After a few months in a cooler, a body will experience some dehydration.

Technicians working at the coroner's office brought in Laci's body first. Both bodies were wrapped in plastic with scotch tape.

Contra Costa County
Coroner's Report

Classification: Homicide/Unknown Means
Decedent: Peterson, Laci Denise
Date of Death: April 14, 2003—Found
Time of Death: Unknown

Date of Birth: May 5, 1975
Age: 27
Sex: Female
Race: Caucasian
Height: Five feet one inch
Weight: Fifty-seven pounds
Hair: Brown
Eyes: Brown
Usual Address: 523 Covena Avenue, Modesto, CA
Identified By: California Department of Justice DNA Lab
Next of Kin: Sharon Rocha, Mother
Place of Death: Point Isabel Regional Shoreline Park
Cause of Death: Undetermined

I have performed autopsies on dozens of bodies that have been in rivers and lakes for weeks and months. My first such experience with bodies that had been submersed for long periods of time occurred the first weekend in August 1961. I had just started my forensic pathology training in Baltimore immediately after getting out of the US Air Force. It was extraordinarily hot that weekend in Baltimore, and someone had turned on the fire hydrant in the inner-city streets to let the water pour out so that kids could play. The force of the water was so strong that it knocked one small boy off his feet and washed him down into a drainage area and into the city's sewer system. They found his body several days later.

Just a few days after that, a migrant worker who had been picking tomatoes along the Maryland shore apparently drank too much liquor and fell into one of the huge tomato-processing pools and drowned in tomato paste. I remember to this day what both of their bloated bodies looked like.

In addition, we have three large rivers in Allegheny County, where the Monongahela and the Allegheny rivers join to form the Ohio River. Every year several drownings occur. Sometimes the bodies are not recovered for several weeks or months. And I have seen a number of them.

So I was prepared for a very graphic scene when they brought out the remains of Laci Peterson. The head and neck were missing, as were both arms, one leg, and part of the other leg. All of the internal organs—lungs, heart, kidneys, and liver—were gone. There was no internal soft tissue of any kind, except for the uterus. I have no explanation for that, nor does it raise any issues or suspicions. The most intact portion was the buttock region—the muscular gluteus maximus and gluteus minimus were there except for the overlying skin and subcutaneous, or fatty, tissue.

As I examined the body, Henry took autopsy photographs. He had brought his forensic photographic equipment with him. All I need when conducting an examination is a notepad and an ink pen. I don't fancy myself as a forensic photographer, so I was glad he would do it.

We started at the top of the torso and moved down, making observations as to possible points of injury. We looked at sites where the head was disarticulated from the lower neck, where the arms were disarticulated from the shoulders, and the legs from the pelvic regions. Specifically, we were searching to see whether there were any markings or other evidence that these body parts had been removed by way of a saw or some other cutting device, such as a hand saw or a chain saw. We found no such evidence.

We also searched the body for any evidence of a bone fracture that might indicate a stab wound or a gunshot wound. Again, we found no such evidence.

The coloration of the body was a dull, grayish white to grayish tan, as compared to the greenish black color of decomposed bodies that have been exposed to the air. The skin was completely gone. A small bit of musculature remained. Bodies do not decompose as fast in water as they do on land. A body exposed to the elements on land for three or more months would experience skeletonalization. In a desert situation, a body might undergo mummification. The fact that these two bodies were in salt water also helped to preserve them.

There's also the question of bacteria in the bowel. Bacteria do not simply die the moment a person dies. In fact, bacteria thrive in a dead body. They are also what lead to a greenish discoloration of the abdomen, which can occur postmortem. Now, if the body has been eviscerated and all the internal organs and tissues have been taken out, then there is really nothing to decompose. The skin will become somewhat dehydrated. The smell is due to the bacteria in the gut.

Because of the condition of the body, it was impossible to determine cause of death and time of death. It was clear that the body had been underwater for at least two or three months. But there was no way scientifically to demonstrate that the body had been in the water since the night of December 23 or the morning of December 24, anymore than we could prove it could not have been there before the night of December 30.

While we could not scientifically prove what caused Laci Peterson's death, it was rather clear that she must have been weighted down in the San Francisco Bay. The pull of water currents in the bay caused the body to glide and float under the water, despite being restrained by weights. The weights were not going to fall away because they were embedded with the ropes tied around her arms, legs, and probably her neck. As decomposition took place, the arms, legs, and head pulled away from the joints. It didn't require any breaking of bones because once the overly soft tissue surrounding the joint space disintegrates, the bones will simply pull apart.

Dr. Brian L. Peterson, a forensic pathologist who had conducted the autopsy for the Contra Costa County coroner's office, officially declared the cause of death as "undetermined." The only drug for which Laci showed positive in the toxicology test was caffeine. Dr. Peterson was not related to Scott.

"The absence of body parts in this case may simply be attributable to postmortem change, animal feeding, and tidal action," Dr. Peterson wrote in his report. "There is no evidence of tool marks on remaining bones of the extremities or on the thoracic vertebral column [backbone]."[18]

Four x-rays were taken of the remains. They showed nothing unusual. The autopsy investigative report stated that an underwire brassiere was attached to the torso by two hook-and-loop-type fasteners. Authorities also recovered khaki-colored trousers and underwear with an elastic band.

After Henry and I examined Laci Peterson's body for nearly ninety minutes, technicians brought in the body of Conner Peterson. The baby's body, which was intact, weighed three and one-half pounds. There was no loss of any portion of the baby in terms of limbs or head. The internal organs had been removed during the original autopsy. All of the soft tissue was macerated from decomposition in the water. A thorough examination revealed that there was no evidence of trauma of any kind. There were no skull fractures.

The coloration of the body was the same dull whitish gray as that of his mother. But it was clear that the baby had been exposed to the water and currents for a much shorter time period than Laci's body. In fact, it had probably just been a few days.

The biggest issue was the baby's body development. To obtain an accurate estimate of age, we measured the baby's length. Decomposition does not impact length because a person's bone structure does not shrink from immersion. Conner measured about nineteen and one-half inches, which is technically within the range of a full-term baby. Plastic tape had been and still was wrapped around the neck and held there by a knot.

We were impressed by the fact that Conner's remains were much less decomposed than Laci's. The body mass of a baby is considerably less, so the expectation would be for it to decompose much more rapidly if it had been in the water the same amount of time. That told us either that the baby had not been placed in the water at the same time as the mother or that the baby had been inside the mother's uterus, where it had been protected from the water currents, and came out later. In fact, my estimate is that Laci's uterine wall decomposed, leading to the baby's extraction. My belief is that Conner was out of the womb and in the water for only two to five days before washing ashore.

Throughout the autopsy examinations, Henry and I spoke very little. It is not the time or the place to make any comments, offer any analysis, or show any signs of surprise or emotion. If you do want to make an observation to a colleague, you do it in sotto voce, or by quietly pointing a finger or something like that. You have to keep in mind that nothing is confidential in this situation. The prosecutor would not be hesitant to ask at trial, "Doctor, didn't you say to your colleague, 'thus and thus,' and now you're saying something differently." You do not make comments. You do not express opinions. You do not show any great surprise or disappointment at anything. Again, a prosecutor could ask you in front of the jury during cross-examination, "Doctor, did you utter an audible gasp or say, 'Oh my God'?" You have to remain impassive. You aren't there to teach. You are there to conduct an examination.

As we left the coroner's office that day, a mob of reporters surrounded us. Mark Geragos introduced Henry and me to the reporters. He provided them with a few brief comments about our professional and academic backgrounds.

"There's not much that we can talk about obviously between the gag order and just in deference to both the Peterson and Rocha families," Geragos told reporters. "Obviously, Dr. Wecht and Dr. Lee have agreed to come onboard and to help us in this matter. Both are thought of in their fields as the foremost experts. Given the consequences in this case, and given, I think initially at least, some of the investigative things that were done, I think it was important to get the best people in the field."[19]

That afternoon Geragos drove Henry and me to the Berkeley Marina where Scott claimed he had put his boat in the water to go fishing. He then took us a couple of miles away to Point Isabel, where Laci's body had floated ashore. As we stood there on the grassy beach, Geragos pointed to the Bulb, a peninsula that juts into the eastern San Francisco Bay where artwork was displayed that featured satanic worship. Geragos told me that some of the paintings included infants submerged in water with their umbilical cords attached, as well as paintings of a man in a boat beheading a woman.

The next morning we went to the home of Scott and Laci Peterson at 523 Covena Avenue. Someone was supposed to have a key to let us into the house. But either that person had forgotten the key or the key didn't work. What happened next was almost comical in the midst of the tragedy. Henry and I decided to scale the eight-foot wooden fence that surrounds the middle-class ranch-style house in order to get inside. Mark Geragos and his investigator followed.

Henry gave me a boost, allowing me to plant my foot on a horizontal bar of some kind. I then straddled the fence, just as I did when I was a kid climbing into a neighbor's yard to retrieve my football. I put one leg up over the fence and then jumped down on the other side. I hadn't done that in a long, long time.

Now don't get me wrong; we had permission to be there. This was not breaking and entering. No one lived there at that time. For about an hour, we walked through the house. We weren't there expecting to find evidence or hidden blood spatters or a mystery hair. We only wanted to inspect the physical layout of the home. We all became quiet when we entered the room that Scott and Laci had painted and prepared to be Conner's nursery.

Fortunately, we didn't have to scale the fence to leave. We went out the front door.

From there, Geragos took us to the home of an elderly couple in the neighborhood. If you had to cast grandparents for a Hollywood movie, you couldn't do better than these folks. Both were in their eighties, but very sharp and alert. He was a graduate of Stanford School of Law and had served on the Modesto City Council. She was a lovely lady. It was a second marriage for both of them.

The couple offered us tea and coffee. We sat in their living room for at least an hour, having an enjoyable conversation. That's when she told Henry and me that she had seen Laci Peterson walking her dog on the morning of December 24, just as Scott had claimed. There was no doubt in her mind whatsoever that she had seen Laci on the date in question.

I flew home to Pittsburgh the next morning with one overriding thought: How in the world did prosecutors call this a slam-dunk case? Not one piece of physical or forensic evidence connected Scott Peterson to the disappearance and the murder of his wife. Not one blood spot in the house, his car, or his boat. Not one scratch on Scott. No evidence of trauma on Laci.

Because of the overwhelming media coverage, Geragos asked to have the trial moved out of Modesto. Judge Delucchi agreed and moved the trial to Redwood City. Nearly sixteen hundred local citizens were summonsed to jury service. For three months prosecutors, defense attorneys, and the judge questioned jurors about their knowledge of the case in an effort to see if they would be fair and open-minded jurors. Any prospective jurors who said they were opposed to the death penalty were automatically dismissed.

On May 27, 2004, the court and the lawyers decided on twelve jurors and six alternates. There were six men and six women, ranging in age from late twenties to late sixties. They included a former police officer, a local public school coach, a county social worker, and a Teamster who worked the graveyard shift at a warehouse.[20]

Opening statements began June 1 and lasted two days. Prosecutors started, taking the better part of four hours to explain to jurors the state's theory in the case. Deputy District Attorney Rick Distaso portrayed Peterson as a habitual liar who feared that his wife and his mistress would learn about each other. "Ladies and gentlemen, this is a commonsense case," Distaso told the jury. "At the end of this case, I'm going to ask you to find the defendant guilty of the murder of Laci Peterson as well as the murder of his son, Conner."[21]

Defense attorney Mark Geragos said he could only agree that his client's conduct had been that of a cad. "You want to say his behavior is boorish, we are not going to dispute that," he told the jurors. "But the fact is that this is a murder case and there has to be evidence in a murder case."[22]

Geragos asked jurors if they knew how much forensic or physical evidence prosecutors had against his client: "Zero. Zip. Nada. Nothing," he told them. The lawyer then dismissed the prosecutors' arguments that Peterson was "stone-cold" emotionally to the disappearance and subsequent death of his wife and unborn son. "He was very emotional behind closed doors," Geragos said.[23]

Prosecutors presented 174 witnesses during the five-month trial. Scores of tape-recorded telephone conversations between Scott and Amber Frey were played to the jury. There were witnesses who testified that Scott was on his cell phone, chatting and laughing, at the New Year's Eve vigil for his missing wife. And, as it turned out, the person he was on the phone with was Amber Frey.

One of the state's first witnesses was Ron Grantski, Laci's stepfather. He told jurors that he was immediately suspicious of Scott's claim that he had gone fishing on Christmas Eve morning. "I said, 'I think your fishing trip is a fishy story. Did you do something else? Do you have a girlfriend?'" Grantski testified. "He said, 'No,' and he turned and walked away."[24]

But under cross-examination by Geragos, Grantski shocked everyone when he admitted that he, too, had gone fishing at the exact time that Scott had gone.

Just weeks before Laci was reported missing, Scott had used the Internet to research water currents in the San Francisco Bay and had bought his mistress presents, according to a police computer expert who had cracked the Peterson's home PC. An expert with the US Geological Survey told jurors that his study of wind and tides in the San Francisco Bay showed that if Scott had dumped the body of his wife and unborn son where he said he had been fishing, there was a "high probability" that one or both of the bodies would have washed ashore exactly where Conner's body was found.[25]

Dr. Brian Peterson, the state's forensic pathologist, told jurors that Laci and Conner most likely died on December 23 or 24. He testified that some form of heavy weights or anchors were taped to Laci's neck, arms, and legs before she was thrown overboard into the San Francisco Bay. He said that Laci was probably lying facedown on the bottom of the bay. The currents and tide caused her abdomen to move back and forth over the floor of the Bay. The movement eventually resulted in a tear in the abdomen and a tear in the uterus, thereby causing the baby to be extruded.

That being said, Dr. Peterson acknowledged on cross-examination that he could not determine what had caused Laci's death. "For whatever reason that Laci met her demise, I believe that it was her death that caused Conner's death, that he was still in her uterus," he testified, as jurors were shown photographs of the badly decomposed bodies of Laci and Conner. "If Conner would have spent substantial unprotected time in the water as Laci did, he simply would have been eaten. There simply wouldn't have been anything left."[26]

Dr. Peterson and other state witnesses admitted that they recovered no forensic evidence connecting Scott to his wife's disappearance and homicide. Asked by prosecutors how it was possible for someone to be killed without leaving any physical evidence, the forensic pathologist said that if Laci had been choked or strangled to death, there probably wouldn't be any medical or forensic evidence left behind.

The prosecution's key witness was Amber Frey, the twenty-eight-year-old certified massage therapist who had a four-week fling with Scott Peterson. Frey was called to the witness stand to expose Scott as a cad and a liar.

Prosecutor: At any time, did the defendant ever tell you that he was married?

Frey: No.
Prosecutor: Ever tell you that he lived in Modesto?
Frey: No.
Prosecutor: Ever tell you that he had a child on the way?
Frey: No.[27]

Frey said Scott was extremely romantic and easy to talk to. She said that he got them a private room at a Japanese restaurant on their first date. Afterward, they went to a karaoke bar, where they sang a duet together, danced, and kissed. They returned to Scott's hotel room and had sex. She told jurors that she was worried the next morning that they had slept together too soon, but he assured her it was fine.[28]

Two weeks before Laci was missing, Scott told Frey that he had "lost" his wife. This "would be his first holiday that he would be spending without her," Scott had told her, according to Frey. He told her it was too painful for him to talk about.[29]

Even more devastating were the scores of telephone conversations with Scott that Frey secretly recorded. Prosecutors played and replayed for the jury the phone call Frey had with Peterson on New Year's Eve, in which he laughed and claimed he was in Paris partying. In reality, he was at a candlelight vigil for his missing wife.

"He wants to live the rich, successful, freewheeling bachelor life," Assistant District Attorney Rick Distaso told jurors in closing arguments. "He can't do that when he's paying child support, alimony, and everything else. He didn't want to be tied to this kid for the rest of his life. He didn't want to be tied to Laci for the rest of his life. So, he killed her."[30]

Because the state lacked any physical or forensic evidence linking Scott to Laci's disappearance, prosecutors focused like a laser on mountains of alleged circumstantial evidence—specifically Peterson's conduct and behavior immediately before his wife's disappearance and for the three months following. They played tape after tape of Scott lying—lying to Amber Frey about being married, lying to police about having an affair, lying to his friends about playing golf instead of fishing, and needlessly and senselessly lying to his own parents about being in Modesto when he was actually eighty miles away. Prosecutors did an extremely effective job of arguing that if Scott would lie to his own mother and father about his whereabouts, he would certainly lie about killing his wife and dumping her body in the San Francisco Bay.

The defense spent most of the trial showing how police ignored tips from citizens who said they had seen Laci alive after Scott had gone fishing, as well as tips that could have made others suspects. For example, an Oroweat delivery truck driver called police on December 30, 2002, saying he had seen Laci walking a golden retriever through the La Loma neighborhood. However, the driver said police didn't question him until July 29, 2004, nine weeks after Peterson's trial had started. In all, at least 193 people from twenty-six states and the Virgin Islands called the police hotline, claiming that they had seen Laci alive in the days and weeks following her disappearance.

In addition, Geragos presented evidence to the jury that a pregnant female prosecutor who lived in the same neighborhood as the Petersons called Modesto detectives just a couple days after Laci went missing. The prosecutor, identified only as "Michelle," told police that Laci might have been the victim of mistaken identity because the two virtually look alike.

Strangely enough, the prosecutor, who was the same age as Laci, said she also owned a dog named McKenzie, which she frequently walked in the park where Scott claimed his wife might have been attacked. The woman prosecutor told Modesto police that she had been receiving violent threats because of a case she had been handling. Geragos claimed that Modesto police never thoroughly followed up on that lead of another suspect.[31]

Modesto police also received a tip four days after Laci was reported missing from a former police officer who said that he saw a man with a ponytail forcing a woman into the back of a van just a few blocks from the Petersons' house. The former officer, Tom

Harshman, said police ignored his information until June 2004, when the trial against Scott was already underway.[32]

The conclusion from all these unchecked tips, Geragos told jurors, was that Modesto police decided from the start that Scott Peterson was the killer and thus ignored all other leads and information.

Geragos also tried to undermine the prosecution argument that Scott was on the verge of fleeing to Mexico at the time they arrested him. To prove their scenario, police pointed to the fact that Scott had more than $14,000 in cash when they pulled him over in San Diego on April 18. But under direct examination, Scott's mother, Jackie Peterson, testified that she had accidentally withdrawn $10,000 from a bank account that was jointly in her and her son's names. She told jurors that she realized her error and gave Scott the cash back on April 17, the evening before he was arrested. He probably didn't have time to redeposit the cash, thus explaining why he possessed such a large amount of money, she stated. Jackie Peterson also told jurors that she had told Scott to borrow her brother's driver's license because he was a member of the Torrey Pines Golf Course in La Jolla and Scott would get a discount using his identification.[33]

As the trial neared its conclusion, Geragos and I, in a lengthy telephone conference call, discussed whether I should be called as a witness. We talked about my hypothetical testimony: What evidence or argument would I offer? Would I be able to contradict or undermine any of the prosecution's forensic testimony? And would my testimony help or hurt the defense's case? I outlined for Geragos the specific points that I would make if called as a witness:

(1) There is no way to tell from examining the bodies of Laci and Conner what day or time they died. They could have died the night of December 23, the afternoon of December 24, or the morning of December 27. My educated estimate is that both had probably been dead for at least two months and probably longer.

(2) There is no way to tell from the autopsy how Laci Peterson died. Her body was in such a decomposed state that the cause of death was impossible to determine.

(3) There is not one shred of physical, medical, or forensic evidence that connects Scott Peterson to the disappearance or death of Laci. There were no scratch marks on his body indicating he had been involved in a fight or struggle.

(4) There is no way to state with any certainty where Laci was attacked. Police found no bloodstains from Laci anywhere. A smudge of Scott's was found in his truck, and a few tiny drops were on the white comforter from the couple's bed. Police made a big public deal when they searched Scott's home and seized ninety bags of evidence. But there was not once any mention during the trial that anything in any of those bags provided one piece of physical evidence connecting Scott to the crime.

While all of these were key points in Geragos's defense of Peterson, he had already gotten the prosecution's forensic witnesses to admit all these points on the witness stand. I told Geragos that this testimony was much more persuasive to the jury coming from the mouths of the prosecution's own witnesses than having me state it. As an intelligent and experienced trial attorney, he firmly agreed.

There were also some pitfalls in having me testify. For example, prosecutors would probably ask me if I agreed with Dr. Peterson that Laci could have been strangled to death in her home without leaving any forensic evidence. I would have had to testify that is true. Nor could I have placed any serious doubt on the state's scenario by citing any scientific or physical evidence. That's because the prosecution's case didn't rely on the forensic evidence, since there wasn't any. But, most regrettably, there was very little physical evidence for me to refer to either.

In the end, we agreed that it would be best if I didn't testify. The same decision was made in regard to Henry Lee's testimony.

Two days later, on October 27, 2004, I was asked by Greta Van Susteren to appear as a guest on her Fox News show, *On the Record.* I agreed. That evening I was sitting in a television studio in Pittsburgh when Greta, who I have known for several years, interviewed me live on national television. Here is part of the interview:

Van Susteren: Doctor, when did you get the word that you would not be called as a witness?

Wecht: Mark [Geragos] and I talked a few times last week and then into the weekend. Late Saturday night, we both decided that Mark had enough on cross-examination of the various medical experts, and there really wasn't more that I could do. I could emphasize certain things. It would be nothing dramatic. And as you know, Greta, on cross-examination, there are certain things that I would concede.

Van Susteren: Well, let me ask you some questions about it. What is your opinion? Is your opinion that Conner was born dead or alive? Was Conner born alive, sir?

Wecht: I'm unable to give a definitive opinion. The organs and tissues were so decomposed that microscopic examination did not yield the answer. If we have a body that is reasonably fresh, then we can make that kind of determination. But there is no way to say that the baby definitely was born dead.

Van Susteren: Let me ask you another question, and I don't mean to put you on the witness stand, but I guess I am a little bit.

Wecht: No, it's OK, Greta. Go ahead.

Van Susteren: Can you estimate when Conner died?

Wecht: No, I can't, for the same reason.

Van Susteren: Let me ask you a scientific question. There has been some suggestion that the baby was in the water [out of the womb] for a short period of time. Could you validate that assertion or not?

Wecht: Yes, I would agree. The dead baby was not in the water for three and a half months. No way. The baby was in the water for two days, three days, four days, something like that.[34]

During closing arguments, Geragos told jurors that it was okay for them to find his client's conduct and behavior disgusting. But that didn't mean that he had killed his wife. And he repeatedly pointed out the fact that there was no physical and forensic evidence indicating that he had.

"Maybe the logical explanation for the fact that we have no evidence of her struggling in that house, dying in that house, is because it didn't happen in that house," Geragos told jurors during closing arguments.[35]

"I would love nothing more than to solve this case and point to somebody and say this is who did it," he continued. "I'm not asking you to nominate Scott Peterson as husband of the year. But the fact of the matter is that they have not proved this case, they have not proved that Scott Peterson did anything except lie."[36]

After five months of testimony, the jury spent seven days reviewing the evidence. Twice during deliberations jurors were removed from the panel because of inappropriate conduct or because they felt too much public pressure to reach a verdict. Those jurors were replaced with alternate jurors. In the end, prosecutors got the jury they wanted. On Friday, November 12, 2004, Scott Peterson was found guilty of one count of first-degree murder in the death of his wife and one count of second-degree murder in the death of his unborn son.

A month later, on Monday, December 13, the same jury, after deliberating for eleven hours and thirty-two minutes over parts of three days, decided that Peterson should pay with his life. The death sentence was greeted by cheers from hundreds of local citizens gathered outside the courtroom. I remember seeing on television that the Rocha family was applauded as they left the courthouse, while the Peterson family was booed and jeered. It reminded me of the lynch mobs that gathered outside courthouses in the Old South a century ago. On March 16, 2005, Judge Delucchi made it official, sentencing Peterson to death.

Let me start by stating that I was not overly surprised by the jury's verdict finding Peterson guilty. Still, I believed there was a reasonable chance that the jury would find him not guilty because there was not one scintilla of hard, tangible physical evidence that connected the defendant to the crime. None. Only minor insignificant bloodstains. No murder weapon. No eyewitnesses or confessions. There was no solid evidence indicating when Laci died, where she was killed, or what caused her death. But there was so much animosity and distrust toward Peterson by the public that it became increasingly clear to me that Peterson was going to be found guilty.

In the end, I think there were two key elements that the defense was unable to overcome. First, the repeated lies by Scott undermined everything else he said or did. Second, the fact that the bodies were recovered ninety miles from the Peterson's home yet only a mile or two from the spot where Scott went fishing. There are only two reasonable explanations: one, Scott did it; two, someone else killed Laci and tried to frame Scott. The problem is that there was no evidence that anyone wanted to frame Scott.

That being said, I was shocked and stunned that the jury sentenced Scott to death. I have witnessed many trials where jurors relied solely on circumstantial evidence to find a defendant guilty of murder. However, I had never seen a single case involving exclusively circumstantial evidence where a jury handed down the death penalty. What usually happens is that juries compromise during deliberations. They agree to find the defendant guilty based on the circumstantial evidence, but they do so only with the understanding that the punishment will be life in prison instead of death.

But this jury, it was clear to me, thirsted for revenge. We are all creatures of our own environment. These jurors' identities were known. Their neighbors knew who they were. That community wanted vengeance. The community wanted blood. My feelings were best expressed in an editorial that was published in my hometown newspaper, the *Pittsburgh Post-Gazette*:

Their verdict may be a little too popular for comfort. This jury sitting in Redwood City, Calif., was not deliberating in a vacuum. Fed by a sensation-seeking media, the nation had obsessed with this case for almost two years and feelings have run high. Cheers went up outside the courtroom when the death penalty verdict was announced. They surely echoed across America. One does not have to be an opponent of the death sentence—as this newspaper has been—to wince a little in the face of blood lust masquerading as justice.

The Scott Peterson case, of course, is far from over. It will be many, many years before he is put to death, if he ever is. At the time that Scott was sentenced to death, there were 641 inmates on death row in California. However, it is a state that has executed only ten individuals since capital punishment was reinstated in the United States in 1978.

That being said, I bet that the California Supreme Court or the federal courts will reverse this conviction and grant Scott a new trial. There were so many issues during this case—from overwhelming pretrial publicity and possible illegal wiretaps to the introduction of improper testimony and evidence. One key issue on appeal will be the dismissal of the first jury foreman, Gregory Jackson. A lawyer and a physician, Jackson reportedly asked to be removed from the jury after several days of deliberations. When Judge Delucchi agreed to let him go, Jackson stated that "given what's transpired, I would never know personally whether or not I was giving the community's verdict, the popular verdict, the expected verdict, the verdict that might, I don't know, produce the best book."[37]

To me, it was clear that at least some on the jury felt pressure from the local community to convict Peterson. Some may have been looking to profit from their jury service by signing a book deal. Moreover, it is only under the most extraordinary circumstances that a judge should dismiss a juror during deliberations. In fact, the California Supreme Court and the Ninth US Circuit

Court of Appeals have made it clear that jurors should not be dismissed simply because they are tired or uncomfortable with the pressure.

In the end, *The People v. Scott Peterson*, the trial that had it all, was missing two significant items: any direct evidence linking Scott Peterson to his wife's murder and a courageous jury willing to put aside community attitudes and pressures in order to decide the defendant's fate based on the actual evidence.

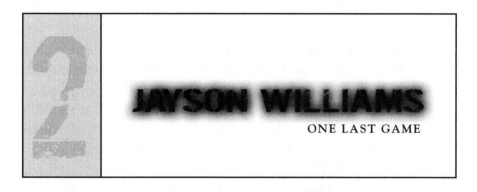

JAYSON WILLIAMS

ONE LAST GAME

Of all the basketball games in which former NBA all-star Jayson Williams had been involved or attended, the one he will probably remember most is one in which he made no rebounds and scored no points. Instead of his New Jersey Nets jersey emblazoned with number 55, he wore Armani slacks and a sweater. It wasn't a championship or even an NBA game. The match took place on February 13, 2002, and Jayson was a spectator, watching America's most famous dribblers do their thing. The night that Jayson Williams received free tickets to see the Harlem Globetrotters would change his life.

Two years later, Williams would take his game to an entirely different court, trying to rebound in life as well as he could on the basketball court.

It was the end of another week after twelve long weeks of trial, and everyone involved was exhausted. The jury was worn-out and the defendant and both families were drained. The lawyers and the judge were ready to drop. Even the television commentators and sports writers were tired of looking for new ways to say the same thing. On Friday, April 30, 2004, the jury reported for duty dressed up a little more than usual. After going through forty-three witnesses and four days of deliberations, this was a fairly good sign that a verdict was imminent. Yet the jurors sent out another note to the judge, fueling speculation as to its contents. One by one the jurors filed into the courtroom. They had reached a verdict.

Both sides had displayed brilliant lawyering. Assistant Hunterdon County Prosecutor Katharine Errickson and Acting Prosecutor Steven Lember relentlessly challenged, objected, and maneuvered around the courtroom. In spite of mass media coverage with cameras allowed inside the courtroom, Superior Court Judge Edward Coleman kept the courtroom under control, not an easy task during a high-profile trial. The defense often felt he was one-sided, but it is likely that the prosecution felt the same way when several of his rulings dealt them heavy blows. He seemed composed and determined to play an impartial role. This was not a tidy little case from *Perry Mason* or *The Practice*, and, as usual, life did not imitate the art of a crime novel.

From college to the pros, and then as an analyst for NBC, Jayson Williams was accustomed to the spotlight and loved it. He was charming, talented, and good-looking. The camera loved him and he had a quick wit. But he had never been in a spotlight like this one before.

Joseph Hayden led the defense team with Billy Martin, with whom I had just worked on the Chandra Levy case. This amazingly solid group consisted of nine expert witnesses and five accomplished attorneys. Other attorneys for the defense included Michael Kelly, formerly a member of the Supreme Court of the state of New York, Chris Adams, and Shawn Wright. Dr. Jo-Ellan Dimitrius, known for her work in other high-profile cases, such as O. J. Simpson, Reginald Denney, the McMartin preschool case, and Scott Peterson, served as jury consultant for the defense. Judy Smith—a consultant in the investigations of the Iran-Contra affair, former Washington, DC, mayor Marion Barry, President Clinton in the impeachment hearings, and the Chandra Levy case—served as communications consultant. Also brought in to testify on forensic matters was my good friend Michael Baden, internationally known for his skills as an expert witness and as a forensic pathologist. Registered professional engineers John T. Butters and Richard N. Ernest were brought in for their expertise on firearms. Forensic toxicologist Dr. Robert Middleberg, forensic pharmacologist Dr. Russel Rockerbie, and forensic psychologist Dr. Joel Dvoskin were all brought in as consultants for the defense as well.[1]

Now, two years and two and a half months after the shooting of Costas "Gus" Christofi, Jayson Williams waited to see if this exceptional team would pay off. Although money may not buy a not guilty verdict, it can pay for the best attorneys available—people who know the law and are devoted and able to thoroughly protect their client's constitutional rights.

Williams knew that he needed that level of knowledge and passion. He was facing charges of aggravated manslaughter, reckless manslaughter, and six other charges stemming from the shooting of limousine driver Gus Christofi and the subsequent alleged cover-up during the early morning hours of February 14, 2002. Now he would find if his lawyers had been successful in proving to the jury that it was a "horrific, totally unforeseeable accident," as defense attorney Billy Martin claimed in his opening statement.[2]

"All right, we will ask you to stand and we will take the verdict from you, Mr. Foreman," Judge Coleman directed Andrew Clark, the foreperson of the jury.

Jayson Williams, former center and power forward for the New Jersey Nets, turned, clasped his wife's hands, and then stood to his full height of six feet ten inches. He was wearing a well-tailored gray suit with a diamond cross in his lapel, a gift from his wife that he'd worn throughout the trial. She said on her Web site about the trial that the cross was something he often wore to depict his beliefs. His Catholicism hadn't harmed his image in the public eye. In his autobiographical book *Loose Balls*, he often writes of his faith, telling how it faltered after watching his two sisters die of

AIDS.[3] News coverage during the trial included stories of his after-church visits to Mr. Christofi's grave, his graduate classes in divinity school, and his weekly Bible studies at his home.

Although he had exhibited a definite grasp of the seriousness of his situation throughout the trial, Williams had not appeared nervous. He took notes on a legal pad, maintained an interest in the arcane legal procedures, and whispered with his lawyers as testimony was presented. His ease and charm with the public showed through as he occasionally gave a juror his handsome smile. As he stood waiting for the verdict, he was still relatively calm, but far from relaxed. His slight side-to-side rocking was quite reminiscent of a ball player gaining composure before a big free throw, but this was bigger than any game he had ever played. This would decide how he would spend the next fifty-five years of his life.

I never saw Jayson Williams play ball. Though I am a sports fan, there is no NBA team in Pittsburgh, and I don't really watch sports on TV. I prefer to enjoy games in person and hold season tickets to the Steelers and the Pirates. I happened to read about the case in the papers, but I did not follow it closely, and, for that matter, I don't remember that it was reported at first in great detail. But, through reading the newspaper coverage, I did recall the fact that he had been a top-notch professional basketball player who had retired early because of an injury.

At the time, I knew the basic facts of the case and would learn other details later. On the evening of February 13, 2002, Jayson went to the Harlem Globetrotters' game at Lehigh University in Bethlehem, Pennsylvania, with several friends, his father, and his nephew. Then, in keeping with his hospitable nature, he invited the Globetrotters to come out to dinner with the group after the game. As a boy, his mother had taken him to Globetrotters games for his birthdays. This had helped him foster an early love for basketball.

Now Jayson was able to repay the team that he had loved as a child by inviting them out for steak and lobster. Four of the Globetrotters met Jayson and his friends at the Mountain View Chalet Restaurant, an upscale family restaurant in Asbury, New Jersey. Jayson had asked his good friend Kent Culuko to phone 78 Limousine for a van to pick up the players who were stranded at the hotel owing to a broken-down bus. Jayson's father and nephew went home. Because of the lateness of the hour, only four Globetrotters took him up on his offer—Benoit Benjamin, Chris Morris, Howard Paul Gaffney, and Curley "Boo" Johnson.

The pleasurable evening out was gratifying to the Globetrotters, who do not get nearly the salaries that NBA players make. (In his ten years in the NBA, Jayson earned $100 million, a remarkably lucrative salary at that time.) Still, it was a typical generous gesture for Williams, who considered himself a blessed man and liked to share his wealth. In addition to making huge charitable donations of money and time, both anonymously and in his name, he had been known to walk into a Manhattan bar with buddies and buy the house rounds of drinks and hand out thousands of dollars to fans,[4] or to walk down the street at Christmastime, giving $100 bills to the homeless who were trying to keep warm on the subway grates.[5]

That night the bar tab for the ten men, including expensive cigars and shots of liquor, was approximately $630 out of a total bill of $1186.30. When pundits argue about the huge number of drinks that this must have covered, they should take two things into consideration. Some of these shots, including Louis XIII Remy Martin Cognac, were very expensive, which later led Globetrotter Paul Gaffney to testify that he was shocked when a couple of the guests drank shots at $100 to $150 a piece. And these were not average-sized men. Jayson, who was thirty-four at the time, was a well-built six feet ten inches and weighed 245 pounds. Given his size and what he admitted was his considerable drinking experience, he was obviously going to be able to hold more liquor than the average man. Later court testimony by wait-ress Margaret DeMatteo, however, reveals that he was by no means the heaviest imbiber of the group, having ordered Chardonnay, espresso, and Johnny Walker Blue.[6]

The group went back to the Williamses' home after dinner. He gave them a late-night tour of his impressive estate, a place he took considerable pride in. While showing off his gun collection in the bedroom, a gun discharged, killing the chauffeur who had been hired for the night. Police and emergency crews were called in.

Nine days later, Judge Ann R. Bartlett signed a complaint war-rant on February 22, 2002, charging Jayson with reckless manslaughter. This is a second-degree crime, carrying a maximum of ten years in prison with a presumptive sentence of seven years. Prior to the grand jury presentation, this was the only charge levied against Jayson relating to the shooting and the ensuing events. Jayson turned himself in three days later and was released on $250,000 bail.

On March 11 additional charges involving tampering with the evidence and witnesses were filed against Williams and two others who were in the house at the time of the shooting. Kent Culuko and John Gordnick later turned state's witness in exchange for plea agreements.

The warrants issued by Judge Bartlett in regard to tampering were for conspiracy to obstruct the administration of law, hin-dering apprehension, tampering with a witness, tampering with evidence, and fabricating physical evidence. Indictments were returned by the Hunterdon County Grand Jury on May 1, 2002. New charges of aggravated assault by pointing a firearm at or in the direction of Mr. Christofi, possession of a weapon for an unlawful purpose, and aggravated manslaughter were added. The latter can carry a prison term of ten to thirty years with a presumptive, or likely, sentence of twenty years.

The differences between aggravated manslaughter and reckless manslaughter would later on prove quite significant. Under New

Jersey law, aggravated manslaughter means that death is brought about under circumstances showing obvious extreme indifference to human life. The jury has lower standards to meet with the charge of reckless manslaughter in that it simply means a death caused by recklessness. To clarify the distinctions, Judge Edward Coleman issued thorough instructions to the jury at the end of the trial: For the jury to convict Jayson Williams on either aggravated manslaughter or reckless manslaughter, it had to find that he was reckless because of a "failure to perceive" that his actions could cause death. To find Williams guilty of aggravated manslaughter, the jury also had to decide that his actions showed "an extreme indifference to human life."

Jayson was arraigned on the first indictment on June 7, 2002. In October the defense asked that the charges be dropped. Williams had cited his Fifth Amendment right to avoid self-incrimination during the investigation. His lawyers claimed that the prosecution had violated those rights by letting the grand jury know of that fact. A future hearing was granted. The prosecution did not wish to risk having its original indictments thrown out altogether, so, in turn, the prosecution filed its own motion, requesting that the first indictment be thrown out and a second arraignment be granted.

On March 10, 2003, Judge Coleman dismissed the original indictment. A new indictment was handed down March 20 for a second set of charges.

Besides all the criminal charges filed, on October 30, 2002, Christofi's brother and sister filed a wrongful death civil lawsuit. This was settled in February 2003 for an amount reported to be $2.75 million.[7]

I did not meet Jayson in person until the fall of 2003. I flew into New York on the evening of September 30, 2003, to meet with Michael Baden and Linda Kenney in their Manhattan apartment, across from the Museum of Modern Art. Linda, an outstanding trial lawyer practicing in New Jersey, was one of the first attorneys called in by the defense. She is quite successful and has worked on cases with Barry Scheck, Johnny Cochran, and others. Her husband, who is the well-known forensic pathologist Dr. Michael Baden, worked with me on the Chandra Levy case. Both are good personal friends of mine, and we have worked together on many cases. Michael had already been brought in as an expert when Linda asked me to become involved in April 2003. Linda and Michael both remained active throughout the criminal trial, but since her husband would be testifying, Linda, as a matter of ethics, chose to avoid any appearance of impropriety and did not attend the trial.

One of the other defense attorneys, Michael Kelly, a former senior assistant district attorney for Buffalo, New York, joined us for a conference there. Mike Kelly is also a close personal friend of Michael's and Linda's and is a fine defense attorney, having tried many homicide cases as a prosecutor. I had worked with him before and knew him from the American Academy of Forensic Sciences. We had a long conference discussing the case at their home and talked over everything. I spent the night with Michael and Linda so that we could get an early start the first thing in the morning. There was a full day of work ahead of us.

Together, the four of us drove across the Hudson River, toward the Pennsylvania line, to the Williamses' home in Alexandria Township, New Jersey. There we met with Jayson's personal attorney, Joseph Hayden of New Jersey, and with Billy Martin, who had been brought in a few months after the case began. I knew Hayden from the Amy Grossberg case (the accused murderer of her newborn baby). Billy Martin was a prosecutor before he went into private practice and was well known for obtaining the drug conviction of former Washington, DC, mayor Marion Barry.

Much has been made of the sixty-five-acre "Who Knew?" estate, which, in truth, is absolutely incredible. Jayson gave the estate its whimsical name because "who knew?" that a boy from the rural south and then Manhattan's Lower East Side would ever have his own private playground? The home is impressive. It is a thirty thousand-square-foot mansion with sixteen bedrooms. The estate includes a lake, a nine-hole golf course, a ten-seat leather-lined movie theater, indoor and outdoor swimming pools, a skeet shooting range, and, of course, indoor and outdoor basketball courts. It is a working farm, designed and built by Jayson and his father, building contractor Elijah Williams. The barn is a working barn that also served as a garage for Jayson's antique car collection—three vintage cars he had restored with his father. Jayson was proud of the place and loved having people over to enjoy it, from friends and acquaintances to underprivileged children.

Jayson's wife, Tanya Young, practices entertainment law with an office in Manhattan and she met with us at the house. She was pregnant at the time with the girl she would give birth to in April 2004, as the trial was nearing an end. They were already parents of a baby girl, and Jayson also had adopted his late sister's two children when she died, one of whom had made him a grandfather when he was twenty-seven.

We sat at a round table in a conference room downstairs. Tanya laid out some sandwiches, salads, and drinks. We had a two- or three-hour work session before Jayson came home. It struck me then, and subsequently every time I met with her during the trial, how absolutely devoted Tanya was to Jayson. She was a real support to him. A lovely woman, she seemed quite involved throughout the trial out of her own choice, sitting beside him in court and working very hard on his behalf, even in the last stages of her pregnancy.

While we were meeting around the table, Jayson walked in. Even though you know someone is a former professional basketball player, the size is still an impressive sight. He gave us all hearty handshakes and seemed a very friendly person. They were a gracious, down-to-earth couple. Anyone would have immediately liked them and, indeed, that is exactly the kind of reputation he has—that of a very affable person.

As much as I enjoyed their company and as lovely as I found the surroundings, I must add that, as a scientist, my mission always is to analyze forensic fact. An objective analysis depends only on available evidence. Still, attorneys present further information, such as personality and lifestyle, to the jury as indications of what kind of person the defendant really is.

Jayson's life certainly provided plenty for the jury and media to examine. The sports columnists that covered him genuinely liked him. The New York Photographer's Press Association awarded him its 2000 "Good Guy" Award. Adrian Wojnarowski, a frequent contributor to ESPN.com and a columnist for the *Bergen (NJ) Record*, wrote that Jayson Williams was the kindest-hearted athlete he ever covered, who had the greatest appreciation for people.[8] Gus Christofi, a working man, was the kind of man Jayson connected with. Indeed, as a card-carrying member of the bricklayers union, Jayson was certainly unique in the NBA. Jayson, wrote Wojnarowski, wasn't "a big famous ballplayer living a life of entitlement and finally getting burned for it."[9]

As mentioned, Jayson was known for his generosity with time and money, publicly and behind the scenes. He hosted basketball camps for underprivileged kids, donated $2.1 million to his alma mater, St. John's University, and gave $20,000 to part-timers at the arena who were laid off during an NBA labor lockout. He heard of a boy whose wheelchair was stolen and replaced it with a better one. He started a foundation to raise money for children with AIDS. All of the money from his best-seller, *Loose Balls*, was donated to Parkinson's research, the disease afflicting his mother. Indeed, to echo David Aldridge in a column for ESPN.com, Gus Christofi was not the only victim of this tragedy.[10]

Jayson Williams was born in rural Ritter, South Carolina. This was the home of his Protestant, African American father, known as E. J. "Big Daddy" Williams, a building contractor with eight children. His mother, Barbara Mazzeo, a Caucasian hospital worker from New York City, was a devout Italian Polish Catholic. They had a farm where Jayson did typical farm chores and had a pony named Mac.

He experienced quite a cultural change at age nine when the family moved to the Lower East Side of New York so that the children could get a better education. "I think they decided the school system [in Ritter] wasn't producing no Rhodes scholars, so we moved back to New York City," he wrote.[11] The streets toughened him up a bit. Playing ball for Christ the King Regional High School enabled him to get offers from several colleges. He cheated on his SATs to get accepted into St. John's University, where for two years his game was on and off.[12] He finally began to consistently play to his potential his third year, leading to a first-round draft pick in 1990 by the Phoenix Suns. He was quickly sent closer to home with the Philadelphia 76ers where he kept the bench warm and the barstools hot for two years. The New Jersey Nets, not doing so well themselves, picked him up. It took a few years for Jayson to get serious about his game, but once he did, he became one of the league's leading rebounders. He became an NBA all-star in his contract year and was signed to a six-year, $86 million contract—at that time, the largest in Nets' history. "I got a big contract in 1998," Jayson wrote, "because I'm a good citizen, and a good teammate, and because I don't do some of the wild stuff I used to. But mostly I got that money because I rebound, because when that ball goes up, I go up too, and I get it."[13]

This was obviously a bright and successful couple. Tanya had her career as an attorney and Jayson his career both as a player and then, after an injury forced early retirement, as a commentator for NBC Sports, where he used his talent for one-liners. Still, the two remained very unpretentious and straightforward. When I met them, they had a definite recognition of the seriousness of the situation. No one was taking this lightly, and no jocularity surrounded our meeting.

At the time, we discussed strategy in the case and the progress of our analyses. Dr. Baden had already done his analysis of the case and of the autopsy. I had done an initial review and had presented the first of several reports in May 2003. We went over the autopsy performed by Chief Medical Examiner Steven Diamond, crime scene photos, postmortem protocol, and the crime scene reconstruction by the New Jersey State Police. We reviewed the report of the state's proffered expert, John Brick, and went over other various reports as well as the transcript of the 911 call placed by Jayson's half brother, Victor. We examined the decedent's clothing and watched a videotape of the scene. We also reconstructed the scene with Jayson.

We toured the house with him to get a feeling for what had happened that evening. He showed us the basketball court where John Gordnick and his two children, along with John McPartland, had been playing ball at the time of the shooting. We saw the recreational room where some of the group had been before and then after the shooting.

Seeing the size of the bedroom in person was very helpful. The judge ruled against allowing the jury to tour the Williams home. This was a shame because pictures and a video tour alone cannot adequately portray how easily that many tall men could fit into the room with no crowding. In a standard bedroom, several men over six feet tall would be elbow-to-elbow and could easily see everything going on and give a fairly accurate testimony. This room contained a table and chairs, an armchair, exercise equipment, an armoire, a gun cabinet, and a bed, and it still had plenty of space in which to move about. Being there enables one to more clearly see how Christofi could have entered the room without Jayson's knowledge. One can also better understand how the testimony of even those who were there could be misstated.

Michael Baden, Linda Kenney, Mike Kelly, Billy Martin, Joseph Hayden, and I watched in Jayson's bedroom as Jayson demonstrated what took place the night of the shooting. The entire reenactment upstairs, complete with our questions, took thirty to forty-five minutes. There really was not a great deal to tell.

Jayson enjoyed skeet shooting and had a collection of six guns in a locked gun cabinet in his bedroom. When Barbara Walters interviewed him about the incident on *20/20*, Jayson said he kept them in his room because that was the safest room in the house. Negative comments have been made regarding this choice. Though I am not a gun owner, his decision makes sense to me. Responsible gun owners lock their guns away in appropriate cabinets, and many choose to keep their cabinet where they can get to it in the middle of the night: in the bedroom. This is the most private room of the house, away from children and away from public display. In my opinion, these precautions of placement in addition to a locked cabinet go to the opposite of negligence. In agreement with the court, he turned over his collection. He says that he no longer shoots or keeps guns in his house.

However, Jayson told us that in the early morning hours of February 14, 2002, he was standing at a particular point in his bedroom with several guests standing around; others were in the adjacent study. He had a lifelong love of guns, one he shared with his father. During this grand tour he was removing each of the six guns from the cabinet and showing them to his visitors. In the trial, friend Kent Culuko and Globetrotters Benoit Benjamin, Chris Morris, and Howard Paul Gaffney testified to being in the room. Globetrotter Curley "Boo" Johnson and Williams's friends Dean Bumbaco, Craig Culuko, John McPartland, and John Gordnick testified that they were elsewhere. Jayson removed the Browning Citori 12-gauge, a top-quality double-barreled shotgun that is popular with skeet shooters. It does not use bullets but shotgun shells, which are full of pellets. Holding it in his large right hand, it took no great effort for a man of his size and familiarity with guns to spin it in an upward motion in order to snap the barrel shut. The gun discharged. Twelve pellets sprayed into Gus Christofi's chest. He collapsed, dying almost instantly.

The two had never met before that night. There was no animosity, nothing negative going on between them. There was no basis for Jayson to have wanted to kill Mr. Christofi. Gus was simply the chauffeur he'd hired to drive the Globetrotters that night. There was no question that this was an accident.

The chief county medical examiner, Prosector Dr. Steven Diamond, performed the autopsy at 8:30 on the morning of February 15, 2002. It was later brought out in trial that Dr. Diamond is not a board-certified forensic pathologist.[14] W. E. Uhlman, MD, and Daksha Shah, MD, both deputy medical examiners, and Sally Cooke assisted in the examination. Also present were three officers with the New Jersey State Police force and a detective with the Hunterdon County prosecutor's office. The death was declared a homicide from a shotgun wound to the thoracoabdominal region (or the upper abdominal area), in the intermediate range. Homicide is a legal term and, under New Jersey law, does not indicate intent. The toxicology report, a routine test for any toxic substances in the body, came back negative. Dr. Baden and I both did separate reports later on the autopsy and we found no real argument with the autopsy itself. Our main objection was that the emergency medical personnel pronounced Christofi dead at 3:28 AM and the body was not taken to the office of the medical examiner for twelve hours. This is highly unusual and disrespectful and possibly can interfere with forensic evaluation.

Mr. Christofi was fifty-five, a recovering alcoholic, and a former drug addict. In the report, it was obvious that his body showed the ravages of the lifestyle that he had struggled successfully to overcome. His years of drinking were the most likely cause of cirrhosis of the liver. X-rays showed that his right hip had been replaced. He had dermatitis, a skin condition, of the ankles, and he was suffering from arteriosclerotic vascular disease and arteriosclerotic coronary disease. These are coronary diseases caused by aging and lead to hardening of the arteries. Not surprisingly, the shotgun wound caused hemopericardium and hematoperitoneum, which means that there was blood in the sac surrounding the heart and in the abdominal cavity.

Gus was a short man, and somewhat heavy. He was five feet five inches tall, or 165 centimeters, and weighed approximately 180 pounds. The shotgun wound was 11 centimeters right of the midline and 11 centimeters below the right nipple, between ribs seven and eight. This left a hole between the fourth and fifth button of his green shirt, about 107 centimeters, or 42 inches, from the floor.

The shotgun wound went right to left and took a slightly upward trajectory. For the wound to take an upward trajectory, this would obviously require that the muzzle of the weapon be lower than forty-two inches, or three and a half feet, the height of the entrance wound, at the time of discharge. Consider the height of a yardstick and add six inches. At six feet ten inches, this would be approximately the height from the floor to the end of Jayson Williams's long arms. Now, take into account the significant difference in height between Jayson Williams and Costas Christofi, along with the length of Jayson's arms. For the muzzle to be less than forty-two inches from the ground, at eighty-two inches in height, Jayson's arms had to be fully extended to his sides. This would be consistent with the defendant's claim that he was holding his arm relatively straight with the gun down by his side, rather than pointing it outward toward Christofi, as claimed by the prosecution. Jayson's stance, with arms fully extended by his sides, is the way one would be likely to stand while snapping shut the barrel of a gun in a swift upward motion.

Dr. Diamond would later attempt to show in his testimony that Christofi was in a defensive position with his arms somewhat raised in protection. The judge dismissed the theory as Diamond's opinion, not based on evidence or scientific fact.[15]

A finding that substantiated Jayson's claim that Christofi had his arms by his side is the blood spatter evidence. Upon reviewing all of the evidence, including the crime scene reconstruction, the autopsy report, and the reports of Dr. Baden and the state's proffered expert, Dr. Brick, I submitted my report to the defense. The fairly discreet pattern of blood spatter revealed in photos was consistent with the conditions of a shotgun wound to the right chest and with the nondefensive posture of a man who had just walked into the room, just as the defense had contended.

The nature and conditions of these spatters also indicated that if, as the state asserted, there had been immediate attempts to place the stock or trigger mechanism into the decedent's hands, the still-liquid blood in these spatters would have been distributed over portions of the hand. This would have caused smudging. There was no such smudging in the photographs.

New Jersey State Police Det. John Garkowski, one of several witnesses to the autopsy, removed the bags that covered Christofi's hands to protect any potential evidence. These bags should always be paper since plastic bags can cut off all the air and might lead to physical-chemical changes of blood and/or other materials. We reviewed the pictures that were taken during the autopsy and saw that the right hand was curved slightly inward with blood spatters on the thumb, index finger, and palm, as well as part of the small finger, or pinkie. On the third fingertip, the blood was smeared, as opposed to being spattered. These smears vary by definition from smudging, which was not found. Smudging would be found on a different part of the hand from the spatter. For example, if you had chocolate syrup on the hands and then wiped the hands on a shirt, it would create a smudge. If anyone had tried to place a gun in Mr. Christofi's hands, blood would have been smudged to other parts of the hands, perhaps from the fingers to the palm or wrist. A blood smear would be at the location of the spatter. On the left hand, the only blood was on the medial aspect of the hand and the medial aspect of the small finger. (Medial always means closest toward the midline of the body when the body is facing forward with the arms down and the palms facing frontward.)

Dr. Baden planned to show the jury that the DNA evidence was not in agreement with the testimony of witnesses who had claimed that Jayson had wiped his prints from the gun. Baden also wished to testify as to whether Christofi was moving before he was shot. In spite of Dr. Baden's forty-seven years of experience as a medical examiner, the judge said these were areas in which the doctor was out of his arena of proficiency and experience, and, moreover, was late in submitting reports to the prosecution. Therefore, he ruled this evidence inadmissible.

I also found that, upon review of photos of the wound, Christofi's clothing, and photographs of subsequent test-firing patterns, the clothing showed the muzzle of the shotgun to be approximately two to three feet away from Mr. Christofi's chest. This, of course, concurs with Jayson's claims that he was not aware that Christofi had walked into the room. In this, Dr. Baden and I found we were in disagreement with the state's expert, our good friend, the well-known criminalist Dr. Henry Lee.

Under cross-examination, Dr. Baden echoed my sentiments when he told of his friendship with Dr. Lee and said that, in this case, he disagreed respectfully. "I love Dr. Lee," said Baden. "I think he's terrific."

During the trial, Dr. Lee would testify for the state that the distance between the gun muzzle and Christofi was six to eighteen inches. A police ballistics expert gave the wide range of one to thirty-six inches. Dr. Baden and I believe that the evidence shows the distance to be twenty-four to thirty-six inches. The importance of these findings is that the defense claims Jayson could not have been pointing the gun at Christofi since he did not know he had entered the room.

To summarize, by reviewing all pertinent information and statistics, Dr. Baden and I found that

1. the distribution of blood spatters on the hands of Mr. Christofi was consistent with a shotgun wound to the chest.
2. the distribution of blood spatters on the hands of Mr. Christofi was consistent with his hands being at his side at the time of the shot.

3. any attempt to place the stock or trigger mechanism of the guns into Mr. Christofi's hand would have caused smudging, which was not there.
4. Mr. Christofi's clothing indicated that the end of the shotgun muzzle was two to three feet away from his chest at the time of discharge.
5. the height of Jayson Williams, the height of Gus Christofi, and the distance of the wound from the floor, along with the wound's upward trajectory of thirty degrees, required the end of the muzzle to be lower than 107 centimeters from the floor. This meant that Jayson's arms had to be extended by his sides, not stretched outward.

Almost immediately following the death of Mr. Christofi, I believe evidence shows that Jayson Williams lapsed into a state of shock. More than one individual in the room noticed his dilated pupils and uncoordinated hand movements. This state of shock is mediated through the autonomic or involuntary nervous system, which results in various physiological changes that reduce blood pressure, thereby leading to diminished oxygen supply to the brain.

The result of this state of shock is disorientation, confusion, bizarre behavior, and other abnormal and seemingly inexplicable behavioral acts. It can even produce subsequent retrograde confabulation (or lying after the fact) and amnesia. All of this was stated in my report of October 1, 2003. Anything Jayson allegedly said or did immediately following the accidental shooting can only be analyzed by taking this state of shock into account. Was he careless and possibly a bit inattentive after the accident? He was quite possibly remiss in some actions, but definitely not in an illicit sense. He settled the civil case for the reported $2.75 million to Christofi's brother and sister. This is right and proper since this tragic accident ended Mr. Christofi's life. But I realized that to turn an obvious accident into a criminal case was absurd.

While we were at the Williamses' home, we also went over Jayson's blood-alcohol level on that night. Much commentary ensued among media members as to why the state did not make a bigger issue of the alcohol consumed by Williams. Court TV anchor Nancy Grace, a former Atlanta prosecutor, insisted every day that she would have centered her case around Williams's blood-alcohol levels. This brings up the fact that as thorough as gavel-to-gavel coverage of a case can be, some things remain behind the scenes. There was a gag order on the case that prevented anyone involved in the case from talking to the press. So press speculation was sometimes simply that—speculation.

Blood-alcohol evidence was not entered into the trial because of the 1923 federal case of *Frye v. US* and the 1993 Supreme Court ruling on *Daubert v. Merrell Dow Pharmaceuticals*. New Jersey follows the ruling on *Daubert*, in which the Court clarified previous standards, set in *Frye*, regarding admissibility of evidence by expert witnesses. *Daubert* admonishes trial judges to act as "gatekeepers" and to do a better job of policing those who testify as experts and what qualifies as expert testimony. It all goes to the admissibility of evidence.

A sample of Jayson's blood for blood-alcohol concentration (BAC) was not drawn for alcohol testing until almost eight hours after the shooting. This is another instance where action was not taken at the appropriate time. The shooting occurred at approximately 2:45 AM on February 14, 2002. Police were aware of possible alcohol consumption by Williams as soon as Christofi was pronounced dead. Blood should have properly been drawn within two hours. Instead, it was not until approximately 10:36 AM that his blood was drawn. This is unscientific and unacceptable conduct during an investigation and negates the value of the evidence obtained.

There was an additional issue tainting the blood-alcohol levels. While we were at the house, Jayson told how he, in panic and shock, consumed a substantial amount of eighty-proof scotch immediately following the shooting. He explained how, understandably, he was completely distraught and "took the bottle to the head," or swigged it, two or three times. It needs to be understood that Williams was home alone with his guests and that this was a rather immediate reaction designed to calm his nerves.

In Dr. Baden's report of May 13, 2003, he told of meeting with Williams on January 26, 2003. To study the effects of Jayson's consumption of scotch on his blood-alcohol level after the shooting, Dr. Baden had Jayson fill an identical scotch bottle with water. At Dr. Baden's request, he chugged the water as he had the scotch that night. By marking the bottle and measuring, we determined that he probably took in four to six ounces per swallow. Therefore, he would have consumed at least eight and possibly up to eighteen ounces of alcohol after the shooting. This would, of course, greatly alter his blood-alcohol level.

The state's proffered expert, John Brick, used what is known as retrograde extrapolation to determine Jayson's blood-alcohol content at the time of the shooting. This method is employed to determine BAC at a particular time and uses given formulas. Using retrograde extrapolation when the blood was taken eight hours after the fact is unreliable and unscientific, particularly when additional alcohol has been consumed. Bear in mind that the legal limit for drunkenness is .10 percent, and in some states .08 percent. In one instance, Dr. Brick worked with a presumed constant alcohol burn-off rate of 0.015 percent per hour. Eight hours times 0.015 percent equals a total burn-off of 0.12 percent. At the time his blood was drawn, eight hours after the shooting, Jayson's BAC was 0.11 percent. Dr. Brick then added the burnt off 0.12 percent to the current 0.11 percent to arrive at the figure of 0.23 percent blood-alcohol level at the time of the shooting, more than twice the legal limit. In short, quite drunk in anyone's book.

However, there are several important issues that Dr. Brick did not take into consideration. He did not take into consideration the immense amount of alcohol Williams had chugged down after the shooting, nor did he take into consideration any other burn-off rates. Some people metabolize their alcohol at the rate of .07 percent per hour. This would change the calculations from 0.23 percent to 0.17 percent, a drastic difference. And if one figures in the additional approximate ten to twelve ounces of scotch, his BAC could have been raised between 0.11 and 0.13 percent after the shooting, changing the BAC at the time of the shooting to between 0.12 and 0.10, using Dr. Brick's calculations. There are other accepted burn-off rates as well, such as 0.01, 0.02, or .007 percent. This means, of course, a wide range of BAC levels are possible using the extrapolation method after this length of time and with this many variables.

In August 2003 the court ordered that Dr. Brick's credentials, the attempt to use retrograde extrapolation, and the blood-alcohol level were all legally suspect.[16] Before the hearing could take place, prosecutor Steven Lember announced that he was withdrawing Dr. Brick as a witness.[17] Dropping this testimony and foregoing entrance of the speculated blood-alcohol level as evidence greatly impaired the prosecution's case.

I rode back to New York from New Jersey with Billy Martin and Joseph Hayden. Billy Martin's associate, the sharp young attorney Shawn Wright, and Joseph Hayden's excellent associate, Chris Adams, rode with us as well. I found them quite impressive. We discussed case strategy on the way back.

Over objections by the state, the court changed the venue of the trial from Hunterdon to Somerset County because of prejudicial pretrial publicity. Jury selection began on January 13, 2004, with more than three hundred potential jurors.

A jury of twelve with four alternates was picked on February 10, 2004. During jury selection, the prosecutor used six of twelve peremptory challenges to eliminate six of eleven potential African American jurors. The original jury pool of 320, twice the number normally called, was narrowed down to a pool of 60; two African American women and no African American men made the final sixteen. This led to an unsuccessful defense objection claiming that the prosecutors had violated the 1986 Supreme Court ruling in *Kentucky v. Batson*, which made it illegal to systematically exclude jurors based on race.

The trial brought the quiet town of Somerville, New Jersey, the kind of excitement it had never known. It had been under the constant eye of the national media since the trial had been moved there from Alexandria Township on October 16. Even the local bakery was selling cookies with the Court TV logo iced onto the top.

The twelve jurors and four alternates sat for twelve weeks in Superior Court Judge Edward Coleman's courtroom. One woman had to leave partway through the trial owing to an illness in the family. The other jurors, however, made it through all the expert witnesses, all the many sidebars, and all the many times they were sent on a long recess while Judge Coleman heard legal arguments and decided on the validity of expert testimony outside the presence of the jury. And thanks to Court TV, the nation had gavel-to-gavel coverage with many viewpoints spouted on the side.

Opening statements took place on February 10, 2004, the same day that the jury was selected. The jury listened to more than thirty witnesses for the prosecution before it rested its case on March 17.

The prosecution called all the members of Jayson's February 13 dinner party as eyewitnesses. The diverse accounts that they offered of the events of the night went to prove the old adage in legal circles—that if one hundred people witness an accident, you'll receive one hundred different stories as to what happened. "Commonly, when someone shoots someone, eyewitness statements can be wrong," Dr. Baden would later testify.[18]

Dean Bumbaco, an acquaintance who testified without a plea deal or immunity, said that he did not witness the shooting since he was in an adjacent study. Craig Culuko, a friend through his brother Kent Culuko, also testified without immunity or plea agreement that he did not witness the shooting because he was with Bumbaco.

Kent was a good friend who had played ball in Europe and had once tried out for the Nets. He pleaded guilty to evidence and witness tampering and testified that he was in the bedroom when the shooting occurred. John McPartland, another European player who had met Williams through Kent, testified without a plea deal or immunity that he was downstairs playing basketball with John Gordnick. Gordnick, who knew Williams several years through Kent Culuko as well and who had brought his two sons along to the game, pleaded guilty to evidence tampering and testified that he was downstairs with his sons and McPartland when the shooting occurred. Former New Jersey Nets player Chris Morris, currently with the Globetrotters, was one of the six guests granted immunity or a plea deal for testimony. He testified on Thursday, March 4, that Jayson had held the gun with his right hand "near the trigger" and that the weapon had fired immediately when Williams had swung it up "in one motion to where it just, just went off." [19]

His rather composed account was in contrast to the testimony of Benoit Benjamin, who was also granted immunity. Benjamin, formerly with the Nets, was currently trying out for the Globe-trotters with a fifteen-day contract. Seated in the witness box, he wore a jacket and dress shirt opened at the chest by several but-tons. Under cross-examination, during his second day on the stand, he seemed to surprise even the prosecution when he said that he saw Jayson's finger on the trigger. He also stated that he saw a shell in the barrel, something he did not share with the authorities until almost a year after the shooting. Attorney Billy Martin questioned his credibility during cross-examination; Martin suggested that he was resentful of Williams's success. Ben-jamin was bankrupt and out of a job at the time of the trial. He had approached Jayson for a job after the shooting. During cross-examination Billy Martin also accused him of extortion as barter for an agreeable testimony. The defense also questioned his ability to look down over the shoulder of Williams, who was only two inches shorter.[20] The defense seemed effective in its attempts, since the jury did not later call for read-back of any portion of Benjamin's testimony.

There was no glimpse of Paul "Showtime" Gaffney's on-court clown persona when he testified under immunity. He said that he was in the bedroom but was walking toward a closet on the opposite side of the room and did not witness the shooting. Gaffney struggled with his emotions as he described praying at Gus's side seconds after he fell to the ground.

The night of the incident was the first time either Gaffney or his teammate Curley "Boo" Johnson had met Williams. Johnson also testified under immunity that he had been nearby but had not witnessed the moment of the shooting. Saying that he doesn't like guns, he asserted that he had walked out of the room during the display and had gone into the study to examine the now-famous bobble-head doll of Jayson. Like Gaffney, he told of attempting to go to the aid of Christofi.

An hour after the prosecution rested, the defense filed a twenty-six-page brief asking for an acquittal on all charges on the grounds that the prosecution had failed to "offer sufficient evidence to sustain its burden." Judges tend to summarily dismiss these rather routine requests, but Judge Coleman set aside the following Monday and Tuesday to hear their arguments. After careful consideration of all opinions, Judge Coleman overruled the request.

Dr. Baden was the first witness called by the defense when he testified on Wednesday, March 24. His testimony was effective and quite powerful in the filled courtroom.

This was also the time that the attorneys had announced they would call me to the stand. I came in around suppertime and had dinner at our hotel with Dr. Baden and the entire defense team. Between the two of us, we could present extremely compelling forensic evidence. Michael had done a thorough job that day, covering all the points and casting doubt on the eyewitness testimony. My own testimony had been saved for rebuttal, but the prosecution did not bring back a rebuttal. Because the defense did not wish to give the state a chance for surrebuttal after I testified, I did not take the stand.

The defense rested two weeks later on March 31, 2004, without calling Jayson Williams to testify on his own behalf. There was no argument as to whether or not the former athlete had been holding the gun. Instead, the case turned into a question of whether the ten-year-old shotgun had misfired because of debris or if Jayson had pulled the trigger in reckless disregard. There had been a lot of long, drawn-out testimony on everything from the bar tab to blood spatters to wood chips in the firing mechanism of the gun.

The very next day, April 1, prosecutors revealed that they had failed to turn over evidence regarding their expert's examination of the gun. In direct violation to an agreement between the parties, the state's expert had taken the 12-gauge Browning apart for inspection with no members of the defense team present.[21] The defense again filed for dismissal of all charges, and again the jury waited.

The trial was suspended until April 15 when Judge Coleman announced that he was refusing to dismiss the charges but was allowing the defense to reopen its case. After calling one witness and recalling four others, the defense rested again. Closing statements took place on April 26, and the case was finally handed over to the jury at 10:56 AM on April 27, 2004.

The jury of eight women and four men deliberated for four days and had sent out several notes during their deliberations. On April 29, after a burst of applause was heard from the deliberation room, the jury stated they had reached verdicts on six of the eight counts but were deadlocked on the other two. Judge Coleman was not about to allow a jury to hang so quickly on those final counts and asked the jury to continue working.

On Friday, April 30, day four of deliberations, Judge Coleman received a note at 3:05 PM. The jury had reached a verdict on all counts but one. Not knowing which count, council for both sides agreed to accept the verdict as is. The twelve jurors filed into the courtroom.

Judge: All right. Have a seat, council. Thank you. And Mr. Foreman we have received your note. We have now marked it as court exhibit C10 indicating that you have a verdict on the majority of the counts but you are unable to reach a verdict on one particular count of the indictment. Is that correct?

Foreman: Correct

Judge: And you feel, for the record, that no further deliberation would be fruitful in reaching a decision?

Foreman: Correct, Your Honor.

Judge: And with that, I've discussed this with council and we've all agreed that what we should do at this point is take the verdict on the counts that you do have. Correct, Council?

Council: Correct, Your Honor.

Judge: So when we go through the jury verdict form, when you get to that particular count, just indicate that the jury has not been able to reach a verdict on that particular count and we will proceed on to the next count. Okay?

Foreman: Yes, sir.

Judge: All right. We will ask you to stand and we will take the verdict from you, Mr. Foreman. [Defendant stands] Will you stand up, Mr. Foreman, please? And the clerk will ask you the appropriate questions.

Each jury member had the following jury verdict form. The court clerk read off the questions and, while the packed court waited, the foreman answered each:

JURY VERDICT FORM
STATE OF NEW JERSEY
V.
JAYSON WILLIAMS
IND. 03-03-00044-I

1. How do you find as to the charge of Aggravated Manslaughter?

NOT GUILTY

2. How do you find as to the charge of Reckless Manslaughter?

UNABLE TO REACH A VERDICT

3. How do you find as to the charge of Possession of a Weapon for an Unlawful Purpose?

NOT GUILTY

4. How do you find as to the charge of Aggravated Assault?

NOT GUILTY

5. How do you find as to the charge of Hindering Apprehension?

GUILTY

If you find the defendant Guilty of this offense, which acts or methods which constitute this offense did you *unanimously agree* have been proven beyond a reasonable doubt?

a) _X_ Destroy or attempt to destroy fingerprints on the shotgun, S-1.

b) _X_ Conceal defendant's clothes worn at the time of the shooting.

c) _X_ Destroy evidence on defendant's body.

d) _X_ Tamper with the location of the shotgun.

e) _____ Tamper with the victim's body.

f) _____ Attempt to induce or cause witnesses to lie to the police.

6. How do you find as to the charge Tampering with Witnesses?

GUILTY

If you find the defendant Guilty of this offense, which acts or methods which constitute this offense did you *unanimously agree* have been proven beyond a reasonable doubt?

a)_____ Defendant told Kent Culuko to say that he was downstairs when the shot was fired.

b)_____ Defendant told Craig Culuko to say that he was downstairs when the shot was fired.

c)_____ Defendant told Dean Bumbaco to say that he was downstairs when the shot was fired.

d)_____ Defendant told John Gordnick to say that everyone was downstairs when the shot was fired.

e)__X__ Defendant told Christopher Morris to say that he was downstairs playing pool when the shot was fired.

f)_____ Defendant told Benoit Benjamin to say that he was downstairs playing pool when the shot was fired.

g)__X__ Defendant told Paul Gaffney to say that he was downstairs when the victim was shot.

h)_____ Defendant told Curly Boo Johnson to say that he was downstairs when the victim was shot.

i)__X__ That defendant told the above listed witness to tell police that all the witnesses had been downstairs when the shooting occurred, which the defendant knew to be false.

j)_____ That defendant told the witnesses that all of them had to make it look like a suicide.

7. How do you find as to the charge of Tampering with Evidence?

GUILTY

If you find the defendant Guilty of this offense, which article(s) has been tampered with, which constitutes this offense, did you *unanimously agree* have been proven beyond a reasonable doubt?

a)_____ Defendant's clothing worn at the time of the shooting.

b)_____ The shotgun, S-1.

c)_____ The body of the victim.

d)__X__ Defendant's body.

8. How do you find as to the charge of Fabricating Physical Evidence?

GUILTY

If you find the defendant Guilty of this offense, which article(s) has been fabricated, which constitute this offense, did you *unanimously agree* have been proven beyond a reasonable doubt?

a)__X__ The clothing the defendant provided to police which

he knew were not the clothes he wore at the time of the shooting.

b)_____ The defendant moved the shotgun, S-1, to make it appear that the shooting had been self-inflicted.

After the foreman had answered "Not guilty" to three of the first four and most serious counts, several cheers were heard from the onlookers. Judge Coleman sternly admonished the crowd and maintained silence for the rest of the proceedings. Jayson hugged Tanya, thanked the jurors, and hurried from the courtroom with his defense team.

When interviewed, jurors said that count two was eight to four for acquittal. Jayson could receive anything from probation to a maximum of thirteen years in prison. Judge Coleman set sentencing aside until a decision on the retrial of the charge of reckless manslaughter was made.

Prosecutor Steven Lember announced on May 21, 2004, that he intends to retry Williams for reckless manslaughter. Upon the request of the defense attorneys, the state appellate division has agreed to review the case based on several issues: Jayson Williams's constitutional protection against double jeopardy; collateral estoppel—a related principle preventing prosecution from reintroducing evidence used in charges of which Jayson has already been acquitted; a six-month delay owing to the illness of defense attorney Mike Kelly, which is requiring aggressive treatment; and the prosecution's request allowing Jayson's prior arrests involving guns to be introduced into evidence.[22] Judge Coleman will not set a new trial date until the appellate division reaches its decision.

After plenty of exercise and practice, Jayson is attempting a comeback in the sport he loves so much. He plays for the Idaho Stampede, a team in the Continental Basketball Association, and hopes to be picked up by an NBA team.

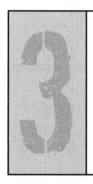

CHANDRA LEVY

LOST AND FOUND

Chandra Levy was scheduled to receive her master's degree from the University of Southern California on Friday, May 11, 2001.[1] At twenty-four, she was bright and pretty, and had a promising future ahead. She moved to Washington, DC, on September 14, 2000, to begin an internship with the Federal Bureau of Prisons. An attractive and vivacious-looking young woman, she had many interests. She enjoyed travel, had been to Israel about a year before with her family, and had worked within the police department during high school. She hoped one day to be an agent for the FBI.

She never made it to graduation.

Chandra's story was not far on the heels of the story of another intern who had left California, come to Washington, and had an affair with a married politician twice her age. Following Chandra's disappearance, a bevy of articles ensued that focused on power-hungry officials and their sexual exploits. The public ate up this tabloid fodder. One has to think that the massive coverage of Chandra's case had more to do with her affair with Congressman Gary Condit than with her status as a missing person. This is evidenced by the fact that there was far more news coverage of Chandra Levy while she was missing than when she was found dead. From the day she was reported missing, her story was in the news continuously until September 11, 2001, when other things filled the thoughts of the nation.

As has happened in too many, less publicized cases, this was a family's loss. A young, intelligent woman with a lifetime ahead of her disappeared. This is a tragic story with some questions that will never be answered.

To understand the mystery of the Levy case, one must grasp the timeline of events.

Chandra spent Thanksgiving weekend of 2000 with her aunt, Linda Zamsky, on the eastern shore of Maryland. She told her aunt that she had an older boyfriend, in his fifties, who looked like Harrison Ford. She finally admitted that he was a congressman and then later let his name slip. A few days before Christmas, she e-mailed a friend, saying that "my man" would be returning to Washington when Congress went back into session. Chandra's landlord later reported that she called him in January about possibly breaking her lease early, so she could move in with her boyfriend. Later, she indicated that it hadn't worked out. Her landlord said he felt that her plans had never really passed the approval of her boyfriend.[2]

The Levys flew from the fairly small town of Modesto, California, in early April 2001, to spend Passover with their daughter, Chandra, and Linda Zamsky, at Linda's home in Maryland. Robert Levy, an oncologist, and his wife, Susan Levy, stayed at a nearby hotel. Chandra, however, stayed with her aunt. It was then that she told her aunt about a bracelet that her boyfriend had given her.

She celebrated her twenty-fourth birthday on April 14, 2001.

Chandra found out that she was now ineligible for the internship she had gotten. The fact that she had finished her actual college coursework early and was no longer active in school disqualified her for that position. Monday, April 23, 2001, was her last day on the job. Chandra left two messages with her landlord on Saturday, April 28, telling him that she wanted to leave Washington, DC, early owing to the early end of her job.

Linda Zamsky got a voice mail from Chandra on Sunday, who said she had something important to tell her. Chandra's landlord also received a call from her Sunday, during which she discussed early lease termination. The next day, Monday, Chandra canceled her membership at the Washington Sports Club and left the gym after 7 PM.

Mr. and Mrs. Levy last heard from their daughter that Tuesday when she e-mailed them information regarding airfares home. Records show that she surfed the Internet until 1 PM.

Chandra's landlord called her Wednesday, May 2, 2001, to further discuss her departure day and received no answer. He followed up with another call and e-mail on Thursday. It concerned him when Chandra, usually prompt in answering messages, did not get back to him Thursday, Friday, or Saturday.

Bob and Susan Levy were beginning to worry about their daughter. That Thursday they called the apartment manager, asking him to open up her apartment to check on her. The manager said he wasn't allowed to do so by law.

By Saturday the Levys were worried enough to call the police. Susan Levy called her congressman, Gary Condit, for help. Apparently, Linda Zamsky had shared Chandra's secret with Chandra's parents by this time, for during the conversation Mrs. Levy asked the congressman if he was having an affair with her daughter. He denied it.

When the Levys told the police that their daughter suffered from severe allergies and could be in need of medical aid, they checked her apartment Sunday. The look around was only a passing one, simply to prove that the young woman was not in her apartment.

Congressman Condit got involved in the case right away. He officially asked the FBI to investigate on Monday, May 7, 2001, and also asked the police department to check into offering a reward for finding her. At the request of the Washington, DC, police, the FBI joined the case.

The apartment manager said two police officers searched the apartment more completely on that Monday or Tuesday.[3] Chandra's suitcases were partly packed and there were dishes in the sink. Her cell phone, driver's license, credit cards, and cash were all still in her apartment. Only her keys were missing.

On Thursday the Levys and Condit announced the reward sum of $25,000 for finding Chandra. The congressman stated, "Chandra is a great person and a good friend. We hope she is found safe and sound." With this statement, he added an additional $10,000 to the reward from his campaign treasury. The *National Enquirer* offered a reward of $100,000 for any information leading to her whereabouts.

As the story escalated, Dr. and Mrs. Levy met for about three hours on Wednesday, May 16, with the Washington, DC, police, the FBI, and a US attorney. The US attorney's office serves in the capacity of district attorney in the District of Columbia. Police informed the couple that cadaver dogs had searched the banks of the Potomac and Anacostia rivers and found nothing there or in the local parks.

Condit had told police in a May 9 interview that the intern was a friend who had visited him at his Washington home. Perhaps in order to quash rumors before they started, he released a public statement: "All of us should focus our efforts on getting her home. . . . It is not appropriate for any of us to make any further comments about the facts of this case or to speculate about a matter that is under police investigation."

While friends and family held vigil in California, The *Washington Post* ran a quote on May 18, by a deputy police chief, saying that Chandra had visited Gary Condit's apartment several times. Moreover, several neighbors of Condit told ABC News that police detectives had contacted them. Police Chief Charles Ramsey later denied the story.

Chandra's Washington friends took up the vigil in her neighborhood on May 19. In the meantime, Condit continued to tell Susan Levy that his relationship with Chandra had been a professional one. At some point in late May, Chandra's parents went through her cell phone records and noticed one number that had been called frequently. Susan Levy called the number, heard soft music, and followed the instructions to enter a phone number. She received a call back from Congressman Condit.[4]

The congressman's so-called professional relationship seemed even more suspect when the *Washington Post* reported on June 7, 2001, that Condit had told police that Levy had, on occasion, spent the night at his condominium. At this point, Condit hired Joseph Cotchett as his attorney to deal with the media. Joseph Cotchett demanded that the *Post* print a retraction on the behalf of his new client, insisting that Condit had never made that statement to the police. When asked if it was true, Cotchett told the media that if Ms. Levy did spend the night at the congressman's condo, she slept on the couch. The *Post* refused to print a retraction.

When the police tried to contact the congressman at his office for a second interview, staffers told them he was not in. Law enforcement officials say that when they followed up with a visit to his home, they were told it was not a good time.[5]

The Levys began to urge Condit to break his silence. They returned to Washington on June 19, 2001, to meet with the attorney they had just hired to help handle their case—Billy Martin, of the Washington firm Dyer, Ellis & Joseph. The following day, Martin announced that his team of private investigators would begin to search for Chandra.

While the Levys were in Washington, Martin arranged for Susan Levy to meet with Condit and his newly hired lawyer, criminal defense attorney Abbe Lowell. Lowell was counsel for House Judiciary Committee Democrats during President Clinton's impeachment hearings. Police, who did not name the congressman as a suspect, interviewed him a second time on June 23. During a third interview on July 6, Gary Condit, a fifty-three-year-old grandfather, finally admitted to an improper romantic relationship with Chandra Levy. The two had first met in November 2000. At the time, Chandra went to his office to meet a friend for lunch, who was an intern for Condit.

Interestingly enough, another attorney hired by the congressman was Mark Geragos—who would soon represent Scott Peterson, also of the small town of Modesto, California.

On July 10 Condit agreed to allow DNA testing and permitted the police to search his apartment. He refused to take an FBI polygraph test, however, which is standard advice among defense attorneys. He was still not named as a suspect, which allowed the police to question him without the presence of an attorney. His attorney later announced that the congressman passed a private polygraph test.

Right before the police searched Condit's apartment again, he and a top aide were seen in Alexandria, Virginia, on July 20, getting rid of a watchcase. Later retrieved by police, this case was traced back to another woman who claimed to have had an affair with the married congressman. Condit did an interview with Connie Chung on ABC News on August 23, 2001. He admitted to making mistakes but would not admit to an affair with Chandra, something he admitted only to the police. He did, however, deny killing her.

While the police and the FBI declined to identify Condit as a suspect, they did investigate the congressman's whereabouts during the time Chandra vanished.

Condit told the Levys that the last day he had spoken with Chandra was the Friday before she disappeared. In contrast, he told police that he had spoken with her two days later, on Sunday, April 29, 2001. Despite this discrepancy, intended or otherwise, it is important to remember that the police investigated the congressman's involvement and interviewed him four times. They stated repeatedly that Condit was not a suspect in the case and found that Condit had an alibi at all crucial times.[6] In addition, after Chandra's remains were later discovered, a Washington, DC, grand jury investigated the Levy homicide and allegations of the congressman's involvement. Documents from Condit's office were subpoenaed, and Mike Lynch, the congressman's chief of staff, was questioned.[7]

Mrs. Condit arrived in Washington, DC, on Saturday, April 28, and was picked up by her husband and a staffer at 7:30 PM. They then went out to eat. This was three days before Chandra disappeared.

Condit's staff said that on Sunday, April 29, 2001, the congressman had brunch, went shopping, and came into the office with his wife. The two went to an Italian market and cooked dinner at his apartment.

Congressman Condit's staff picked him up for work the following morning. He had lunch at the White House and went back to Capitol Hill at 1:30 PM. He left to go home for dinner at 5:30 PM. This was the last day anyone actually saw Chandra.

On Tuesday, the day that Chandra disappeared, Gary Condit's office said that his staff picked him up for work and he had a meeting with Vice President Dick Cheney between 12:30 and 12:50 PM. He returned to the office around 3:30 that afternoon, had a doctor's appointment at 5 PM, and voted on the House floor at 6:25 and 6:35 PM. The Condits had dinner at home that evening. Chandra's whereabouts on that day can be verified until about 1:00 PM, when she signed off the Internet.

Wednesday was the day that Chandra's landlord could not reach her by phone. Condit's office says that he received a ride to work with his staff. He spent the morning in agriculture and intelligence meetings, and then he placed his vote at 11:30 AM. The California congressional delegation met at noon. This was followed by another trip to the White House. The congressman had more meetings at the Capitol beginning at 2:30 PM, followed by another vote at 4 PM. He met with an ABC News reporter at a neighborhood coffee shop at 4:30 PM and had dinner with his wife again that night.

Mrs. Condit left Washington, DC, the next day.

In spite of these alibis and clearance by the authorities in the matter of Chandra's disappearance, Condit's political career was ruined. In an effort to salvage his image before elections, the congressman issued a letter to his constituents the day before his interview with Connie Chung in August 2001. He expressed sorrow at the Levys' pain but said nothing about his involvement with their daughter. He also gave a lengthy interview to *People* magazine. These appearances failed to help. He lost his bid for reelection during the primaries in March 2002. This was after a career of seven terms as the congressman for his district in the Central Valley of California. Guilty or innocent, the public judged him harshly, both for having an affair and for lying about it. In addition, the Levys voiced discontent with his lack of candor, fearing that it may have hurt the investigation and wasted valuable time. His career was over.

When police investigators searched Chandra's computer, they found a map of Rock Creek Park on the park's official Web site, currently http://www.nps.gov/rock/. Apparently, she had done a search for directions to the Pierce/Klingle mansion, which was close to the spot where her remains were later found. Within walking distance of her apartment, the historic stone farmhouse was constructed in 1823 and now serves as headquarters for the superintendent of the park. It is only open for tours on Saturdays and Sundays. Chandra visited the park on a Tuesday. Reports state that the Park Service Department was closed as well. The park itself is open seven days a week except for Christmas, New Year's Day, Thanksgiving, and the Fourth of July.

In spite of several lengthy searches of the park with cadaver dogs, police did not find Chandra's remains. On Wednesday, May 22, 2002, nearly a year and a month after Chandra last visited the park, a man followed his dog off of the general path when his pet began digging in leaves for a turtle. The man discovered the skull on a steep slope less than a mile from Pierce/Klingle mansion. Based on her dental records, the remains were identified later that day to be those of Chandra Levy. Reporters and photographers gathered en masse and were joined by the Washington, DC, Metropolitan Police, the FBI, the Park Service, the Justice Department, and private investigators hired by Billy Martin, who had been brought in by the Levys in June of the previous year. Because of the heavy media attention, the Levy family found out by watching television that their daughter's status had changed from that of a missing person to that of a murder victim. Police investigators did additional searches the following day, hoping to find hair, blood, fiber, or any other evidence to help solve the mystery. Satellite trucks and news reporters, eager to catch some tidbit from the secluded family, surrounded the Levys' home in Stanislaus County. All that there was to report was the sight of friends filing in and out among the old yellow ribbons that mournfully bedecked the neighborhood.

I had, of course, watched the news story unfold over the year like everyone else and found it fascinating in scientific terms and also as a human-interest story. Although I had no specific involvement, I was asked many times to speculate on the search by newspapers and television news programs.

Once Chandra's remains were found, the tragic case entered the media cycle with a renewed force. For the next several days, my schedule was full of interviews with newspaper reporters and radio and television talk shows who wanted my opinion on the case. I received calls from *The O'Reilly Factor* of Fox News, my friend Greta Van Susteren of *On the Record*, CourtTV's Katherine Crier, and MSNBC, to name a few.

Calls of this nature are usually from one of the show's producers. The producer, who nine out of ten times is a young woman, will usually set up a preprogram interview. This is to find out what your take is on a case. They often send wire reports and sometimes even the autopsy report for me to examine. I then do my best to give an educated guess. Sometimes these producers are quite knowledgeable on the subject, and sometimes it is surprising how little they know. It is always nice to find out what the host will ask ahead of time, since it allows me to give more thoughtful responses.

It wasn't long after Chandra's remains were found that my good friends and colleagues Dr. Henry Lee and Dr. Michael Baden and I were brought in by the Levys to offer a second opinion on Chandra's death. While all of us are more than competent in the field of forensic pathology, each of us has his own area of specialty. Dr. Baden is codirector of the New York State Police medical investigation unit; Dr. Lee is the chief emeritus of the Connecticut State Police Laboratory and has investigated more than four thousand homicides. Dr. Lee also happens to be a fine forensic photographer. All of us have served as expert witnesses in court multitudes of times. When Billy Martin recommended us for this case, we agreed to take it pro bono.

Although it is rather unusual for a family even to hire a lawyer when no one is suspected of a crime, it is a very wise move if they can afford it. Attorneys—because of their status in the justice system as officers of the court—can often accomplish things that even the savviest people cannot. Whether it is due to connections or to the trading of favors or to professional courtesy, a governmental agency or police department tends to respond much differently to a letter on law firm stationery than to one from a civilian. The Levy family felt that things were not progressing as they wished and that Congressman Condit was being investigated inadequately.[8] When they brought Billy Martin in at the very beginning, they hired someone intelligent and well connected.

Billy Martin of Dyer, Ellis & Joseph in Washington, DC, already knew of me, partly because he grew up in Allegheny County where I am coroner. When he first contacted Dr. Lee and me, we suggested that he get Dr. Baden involved too.

We met with Martin and another member of his firm, Mike

Dyer, in the conference room of Martin's law office in the Watergate Building at approximately 9:45 AM, on July 19, 2002, just two months after Chandra's remains had been found. Dr. Baden's wife, Linda Baden Kenney, was there in the capacity of consulting attorney. Private investigators Dwayne Stanton and Joseph McCann also joined us. McCann had previously been head of the Washington, DC, homicide division. Stanton had worked for him there.

When we reviewed the remains that day, it was not because we questioned the reputation of the city's chief medical examiner, Jonathan Arden, but because it is always a good idea to get a second opinion. In this particular case, we were not even working in any type of adversarial fashion of defense versus prosecution. We were all, so to speak, on the same side. This is why it was so disappointing that we were unable to receive an autopsy report from him ahead of time. We found him less than helpful, which seemed perplexing. However, with or without appropriate information to go over, the eight of us discussed various aspects of the case that morning before leaving for Rock Creek Park—the scene where Chandra's body had been found.

I am not a computer user. However, the Web site for Rock Creek Park is an easy and informative one to use that gives insight as to why Chandra may have visited both the Web site and the park. Online offerings include accessibility information; online sites of the park's bookstore, Civil War Store, and Revolutionary War Store; and some of the history of the park, which was founded in 1890. There is also a map, making it easier to pinpoint where she was found.

Near the Pierce/Klingle House are several other of the park's main attractions: the Nature Center and Planetarium (which is closed on Mondays and Tuesdays), Pierce Springhouse, and Pierce Barn. Pierce Mill, built in 1820 and the only remaining mill along Rock Creek, is under fundraising operations to become a working mill again. This leads us to believe that Chandra either went to the park to meet someone or to jog along its trails. Since she was dressed to run and was found off of one of the many trails, we can assume that one reason she was there was simply to get some exercise in a pleasant environment in the middle of the city. It was an easy place for her to go, since one entrance was just a couple of blocks from her house.

At 1,755 acres, the National Park System lists Rock Creek Park as one of the largest urban parks in the world. It is a lovely place for picnicking, hiking, horseback riding, and in-line skating. There are facilities for soccer, tennis, and fishing, and a visitor can also enjoy a concert or a program by a park ranger. It is quite picturesque and has much to offer someone who enjoys nature or wants to get away for a short while. The year that Chandra Levy was killed, she was one of 2,131,518 visitors to the park. In spite of this and police searches, not one person came across her remains in more than a year. A trip to the scene, however, showed me how this could be entirely possible.

Visiting this particular crime scene illustrated many reasons for walking through the setting where a death occurred. When possible, it is always a good idea for the forensic scientist to do so. Sometimes you can learn something or gain new insight. It aids in the mental process of reflecting on what might have happened. You never know how different aspects of the case will be tied together. When a shooting, stabbing, or beating is suspected, this approach is almost invaluable. Another aspect is pretrial preparation. When an attorney questions your credibility on the stand by asking if you attended the scene, an affirmative answer helps add to your reliability in the minds of the jury.

The area where Chandra's body was discovered was out of the way and not a place one would go without purpose. We walked on a manure-dotted horse trail through heavily wooded surroundings. To get to the place where her remains were found, we had to climb down a fairly steep hill at about a seventy-five-degree angle. We had to walk very carefully to avoid slipping on the leaves that completely carpeted the ground. An orange stick was hammered into the ground, marking the scene of the police investigation and where her remains were found. Dr. Lee, Dr. Baden, and Linda Baden Kenney took pictures while we discussed how Chandra might have gotten down there. Actually traversing the area ourselves, we reinforced in our minds that it was not an area she would have been casually walking through. It is very steep and difficult to get to. It is not a shortcut to anything and lies between two pathways or small roads. Her parents told us that, while she enjoyed jogging, she was not a hiker or into heavy trekking. Still, too many trees and other obstacles blocked the way for her body to have been pushed or rolled down that incline. A hollowed-out area was on the incline where we believe the body was found, since police stated she was buried in a shallow grave. It is likely that her body was placed there after someone killed her.

About twenty feet below the site where her body was found, there was a large fallen tree, the circumference of a small redwood. This would have made an ideal place for two people to sit in conversation. Farther down the hill was a stream, small enough to be crossed on a few rocks. The second path was on the other side of the stream. Not far downstream from where we crossed on the stepping-stones was another fallen tree. This served as another way of crossing the stream by acting as a natural bridge. We were all out there in dress clothes and shoes, but a young, agile person in sneakers could walk on the tree quite easily. This tree also served as a very good trysting place for two people wishing to hold a conversation in private.

We walked around the site and discussed the possibilities of what may have happened and where. Did the young woman go to this out-of-way spot to meet someone she knew or was she accosted by a stranger? Was she the victim of a rape that became a murder? After examining the area, we realized it was time to meet with Dr. Jonathan Arden.

We had a prearranged meeting at the Washington, DC, medical examiner's office. Billy Martin had spoken with Dr. Arden earlier in the day. It was agreed that we would arrive anytime between 11:00 AM and 2:30 PM. We expected to be there around 11:30 that morning but arrived closer to 11:50 AM. Billy Martin said that Dr. Arden told him that he had things to discuss with us that he couldn't say over the phone. He also let him know that he would open up all his files to help in our investigation for the family. Yet, when we arrived, we were told that Dr. Arden had left twenty minutes before. He had been called away.

This was interesting in that it was similar to the Laci Peterson case. In neither situation was the medical examiner we were dealing with present. These were big cases, and the appointments had been set up for some time. We are fellow forensic scientists and all members of the American Academy of Forensic Sciences. Whether the prosecution or defense engages outside pathologists, and in this situation it was actually neither, we all have the mission of finding the truth and are supposed to be collaborators in that mission.

There was some consternation in getting the whole situation sorted out that day, and this caused an unnecessary delay. Finally, after many phone calls, Eileen, the legal counsel for the medical examiner's office, came down to greet us. She had worked things out and told us we would be dealing with Dr. Marie-Lydie Pierre-Louis, the assistant medical examiner. The two of them led us to the basement at the morgue. An assistant brought out three boxes from Dr. Arden's office. Dr. Pierre-Louis informed us that she had never seen the contents of the boxes or even discussed the case with Dr. Arden. Because of this, she wished us to open and examine the contents of only one box at a time. This prevented us from setting up the entire skeleton at once, a far from ideal situation. Other than this, she did not interfere with our work at all, allowed us to take photos, and was generally very congenial.

We reviewed the remains for about an hour, from 12:15 to 1:15 PM. The three boxes, a large, a medium, and a small, were labeled H-021795. The smallest box contained the hyoid bone and other small bones. The hyoid bone is a two-inch-long, u-shaped bone beneath the mandible, or the lower jaw. It was labeled "Do not release." Seventeen x-rays were available for review, along with two envelopes that contained four x-rays of the long bone. There was also an envelope holding three separate dental x-rays. Only 25 percent of the hyoid bone had been recovered, but what was available to examine would prove to be important in our conclusion.

Dr. Arden, I believe, had given the impression on television that most of the bones had been found. Actually several bones were missing: the ulna bone, which is the part of the forearm opposite of the thumb; the left pelvis, which is quite large; a number of the vertebrae; some foot bones, including one right phalanx; and some ankle bones.

Even though the bones had been open to the elements and wild animals for more than a year, we were still able to learn from them. The skull was darkened on the left side, showing that her head had been lying on that side with the right side in an upright, exposed position. The right side of the face was cracked. Without microscopic examination, it appeared to be postmortem, since we could not see any discoloration or bleeding at the location of the crack. The hyoid bone also appeared cracked, but the end of the fracture was discolored along the fracture line, indicating probable bleeding. Bleeding does not occur after death. To confirm, however, the bone needed to be examined under a specialized microscope. To do so, I would have made a cross section through the bone, examined it, and decalcified it. This process also occurs when a surgeon removes a bone in the hospital to see if a tumor or osteomyelitis (an inflammation of the bone or bone marrow) is present. If the discoloration had been present because of bleeding, iron would have shown up at the fracture line. This is due to the fact that iron is the by-product of the breakdown left on a bone after decomposition.

Doing this decalcification could have helped us determine in a more absolute manner the cause of death. A predeath fracture of the hyoid bone would indicate strangulation. The hyoid bone, also known as the lingual bone, supports the tongue. The bony arch is of horseshoe shape and is in five segments—a body, two greater cornua, and the two lesser cornua. This microscopic examination was necessary for us to see what we were looking for. Taking a slice from the bone would have caused it minimal damage and would not have prevented officials from conducting any essential investigations. The body belongs to the family and, in accordance with the Jewish faith of the Levys, needed to be intact for burial. Although the law of the District of Columbia allows the medical examiner to retain tissues and specimens for further investigation, there was no reason that photographs and slides could not have been used in their place. Instead, we were prevented from doing the exam on the hyoid bone, and Chandra's parents were kept from burying their daughter's remains.

Another finding was also consistent with a violent death. The lower lateral right incisor was chipped in the front. All the rest of her teeth had perfect enamel covering. The tooth next to the chipped incisor was discolored, another indication of bleeding before death. A young woman of this age would not have likely gone long without having a chipped front tooth repaired. This could have been easily confirmed by a look at her dental records, but they were not made available to us.

One of the x-rays showed both femurs together, revealing that the x-rays were not all taken at the same time. While police investigators found the first femur, Martin's private investigators, Stanton and McCann, found the second femur after police had released the crime scene. The x-ray of the two femurs together was likely taken after the initial examination. Again, since no records were provided, I cannot be definite on this matter.

Even this scanty evidence—provided by only an incomplete skeleton examined in separate pieces and through photographs— enabled us to make educated deductions as to the manner of death. She was probably strangled and very likely suffered some sort of blow to the face before death. As in the cases of many other disappearances ending with a body being found, we could not definitively answer who, what, where, or why. The "when" was deduced by records of her personal life rather than by scientific proof.

I don't know what was more painful for the Levys—the months of wondering if their daughter was dead or alive or finding out, after all the months of waiting, hoping, and praying, that she was really gone. Parents and loved ones suffer through this agony on a regular basis. In the high-profile cases picked up by the media, we hear the word "closure" thrown about with ever-increasing frequency. There is no such thing. Perhaps finding that a missing person is dead brings finality to a situation, but I would venture to say that not one family touched by such a situation will claim that they feel closure when their child's body or remains are found.

I am the father of four children and the grandfather of eleven. I cannot imagine the absolute horror, hopelessness, and desperation that would consume my wife and me if a member of our family were missing. Yet in 2001 the FBI's National Crime Information Center listed 840,279 missing person entries. Of these 85 to 95 percent were juveniles. There was fourteen-year-old Elizabeth Smart of Salt Lake City, Utah, who was abducted from her bedroom in 2002 and found alive nine months later. Twelve-year-old Jamie Hicks of Mesquite, Texas, made the news when she was kidnapped by her stepfather in September 2004. The two were found within weeks. Jamie was safe, and he had committed suicide. Everyone knows of the pregnant Laci Peterson of Modesto, California, whose remains were found months after she was reported missing on Christmas Eve 2001. There are many others who never make the news and many whose bodies are never found.

The case of Rachel Cooke, age nineteen, of Georgetown, Texas, near Austin, was similar to Chandra's. Her father, Robert, was a software engineer for IBM, and her mother was a high school English teacher. Rachel was home for the holidays from college in San Diego when she disappeared while jogging on Thursday, January 10, 2002. Eight bodies in or around Williamson County have been found since her disappearance, but she has never been found.

Asha Jaquilla Degree was only nine years old when her father last saw her asleep in her bed in Shelby, North Carolina, at 2:30 AM, on Valentine's Day 2000. The young African American girl has vanished without a trace.

Family members of twenty-year-old Amber Hoopes found the lights and television on in her room at 1:00 AM in Idaho Falls, Idaho. All of her belongings were still there. They had seen her the evening before, September 14, 2001, at 10:30 PM. She is still on the missing persons list.

Architectural design student Cindy Song was twenty-one years old when she vanished after a couple of parties on October 31, 2001, in State College, Pennsylvania. She never reported for work the next day.

Brooke Carol Wilberger of Corvalis, Oregon, was reported missing around 10 AM, on May 24, 2004. Only her flip-flops were found in the middle of the parking lot of the complex where she worked. The nineteen-year-old student at Brigham Young University has never been found. However, right before the publication of this book, a serial killer was charged with Brooke's murder.

Forensic science is better today than has ever been hoped, but it is still not where we want it to be. No matter what levels it reaches, it will never be able to perform magic. We don't know what happened in these missing persons cases, and the chances are we won't be able to tell in similar cases in the future.

Chandra Levy was probably strangled. Still, we can't know, even with all of the knowledge at our disposal, if a stranger accosted her in the park. We don't know if the man, or woman, involved intended a mugging, a rape, or a murder. We are in the dark as to whether she went to the park to meet someone or to be alone, whether her death came at the hands of a stranger or one she thought to be a friend. Like the cases of many other missing persons ending in death, the story of Chandra Levy remains a mystery.

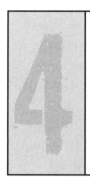

THE CASE OF
JONNY GAMMAGE

DEATH IN POLICE CUSTODY

Jonny E. Gammage was no dangerous felon. In fact, he had no criminal record. The son of a Buffalo police officer and the cousin of a professional football player, Gammage was, by all accounts, one of the good people in the world. He had a place in his heart for the poor and needy, helping them however and whenever he could.

Another thing about Jonny Gammage is certain: he should never have died during a routine traffic stop in Pittsburgh, but that is exactly what happened.

Unfortunately, the injustice surrounding Gammage's death didn't end when he stopped breathing. I believe it is a case that should still be reopened, reinvestigated, and reprosecuted. It is not too late for justice to be served—the evidence is still there. In fact, there may be even more evidence today than there was back then, in 1995. The question is, does anyone have the courage to reopen a case that caused so much turmoil in Pittsburgh nearly a decade ago?

The tragic case began in the early morning hours of Thursday, October 12, 1995. According to initial police reports, a Brentwood police officer observed Gammage, a thirty-one-year-old black man, driving a 1988 Jaguar north on State Route 51—also known as Saw Mill Run Boulevard—at about 1:46 AM. Brentwood is a small, predominately white, working middle-class residential community that borders Pittsburgh to the southeast. Route 51 weaves in and out of Pittsburgh, Brentwood, and several other suburban communities.

The officer, Lt. Milton E. Mulholland Jr., said that he noticed the Jaguar being operated in an erratic manner—slowing, then speeding up, slowing again, then lurching forward. The officer also said the car changed lanes several times.[1]

Suspicious, Lieutenant Mulholland began following the Jaguar for a few blocks. He said the erratic driving continued. Then, according to the officer, the car ran a red light, so he turned on his red and blue lights and siren. Gammage, the sole occupant in the Jaguar, pulled over about a mile from the area where Lieutenant Mulholland first spotted him. Within a couple minutes, four more police officers from neighboring police departments were at the scene of this traffic stop.[2]

Mystery surrounds what happened during the next twenty minutes and why it happened. For reasons that remain unknown, the officers and Gammage started fighting. The policemen forced Gammage to the ground facedown. He was handcuffed. But after a few minutes, someone noticed that Gammage was no longer struggling. In fact, he wasn't moving at all. A paramedic who had just arrived at the scene ordered the officers off of Gammage and turned him over. He checked for a pulse. Gammage wasn't breathing. One of the officers blurted out that he hoped Gammage had died.

At 3:51 AM, Jonny Gammage was declared dead at Mercy Hospital. Gammage's last words before he died were "I'm 31. I'm only 31."[3]

I first heard about the Gammage case when the *Pittsburgh Post-Gazette* and the *Tribune-Review*, our city's two newspapers, landed on my doorstep the next morning. Because Gammage was the first cousin and business partner of Pittsburgh Steelers defensive lineman Ray Seals, the article on the incident was prominently featured on the front page. It was also the lead story on all the local evening television newscasts, dominating news and talk radio stations.

Gammage did not pull over right away, according to Lieutenant Mulholland. But the officer said the driver did not appear to be trying to get away, either. The police originally described it as a "slow-speed chase," whatever that means. They admitted that Gammage never exceeded thirty-five miles per hour. He finally pulled over, they said, in the 2100 block of Saw Mill Run Boulevard, near the Overbrook Elementary School, which is actually back within the Pittsburgh city limits.

According to the officer, Gammage cooperated at first, providing them with his driver's license. He told them that he didn't have the vehicle's registration because the car didn't belong to him—it was his cousin's. Lieutenant Mulholland said everything seemed okay when he went back to his squad car to run Gammage's license and the car's license tag through the police computer system.

For some reason, four additional police officers arrived at the scene and approached Gammage's car. They stated that Gammage refused to obey their orders to keep his hands visible inside the car. They said he also was uncooperative with them when they told him to get out of the car.

"It would be fair to say that at that point, matters began to deteriorate quickly," Brentwood police chief Wayne Babish was quoted saying in the newspaper. "There was a violent struggle between Mr. Gammage and our police officers at the scene. The struggle caused the parties to fall to the ground."[4]

During the struggle, Gammage severely bit the finger of one of the officers, according to Chief Babish. He said the officers eventually cuffed Gammage's hands behind his back and secured his feet with leg irons. The initial police report stated that Gammage went into some sort of cardiac arrest and died.

Interestingly enough, the first newspaper articles about the incident indicated that even the authorities believed there was more to the story than was being told. For example, Chief Babish called it "a very tragic and unfortunate circumstance."[5] He added, "I do expect there will be an open inquest." Allegheny County coroner James Gregris was quoted as saying that Gammage's death occurred under "circumstances that are highly unusual."[6] Because the death had actually occurred within the Pittsburgh city limits, the case was assigned to the Pittsburgh Police Department's homicide division to investigate.

The initial news article didn't discuss the race factor. But being from Pittsburgh, I guessed that Gammage was African American. And I was willing to bet all my money that all the officers were white. I was right. Coming on the heels of the Rodney King beating case in Los Angeles, I knew that this would ignite charges of racial prejudice within the police force.

There is a widespread perception within the black community that African Americans, especially young black men, are unfairly targeted by law enforcement. They believe that their cars are selectively targeted for traffic enforcement. They believe that because they are black, they are automatically suspected of doing drugs or being criminals. For those who say that assumption is nonsense, the evidence shows otherwise. For example, police officers in New Jersey and Texas during the past couple of years have admitted that they selectively targeted black suspects solely because of the color of their skin. And then there are statistics showing that even though white people are the overwhelming consumers of illegal drugs, a great majority of people in prison on drug charges are black.

Then, a case like Jonny Gammage's comes along, fueling the anger, frustration, and bitterness created by those injustices. My gut feeling as I read the first *Post-Gazette* article about Gammage was that the issue of police and racial relations in Pittsburgh was about to erupt.

Two days later the Reverend Jesse Jackson declared Gammage's death "a lynching" at the hands of white cops.[7] Several hundred people marched in the streets. Tensions between the police and the black community were high and rising.

Chief Babish, whom I came to respect because of this case, announced that his department was "distraught" over Gammage's death and that the officers had been placed on temporary medical leave, pending the outcome of the investigation. He asked the public to wait until the probe was complete and the facts were revealed before making a judgment on his department. He repeatedly stated that his thoughts and prayers were with Ray Seals and Gammage's family.

Chief Babish had been the head of the Brentwood Police Department for only a year, but I had been told that he was very concerned about maverick officers who liked to play tough guys. In fact, a lawyer provided me with a memo that Chief Babish had written earlier and sent to his police officers warning them about their conduct.

"The bullying or bombastic Brentwood police officer who believes that a motorist must be given a tongue-lashing for a minor infraction or when an arrest is made, is generally a coward in uniform," Chief Babish stated in the memo.

Jonny Gammage grew up in Syracuse. He was the only son of Jonny L. and Narves Gammage. He had four sisters but no brothers. Jonny and Ray were best friends growing up. Both loved football. Jonny was small, just five feet six inches tall and 165 pounds; while Ray was huge, six feet three inches and nearly 300 pounds. When Ray chose to play semiprofessional football, Jonny decided to go to college full time, graduating from Buffalo State College in 1989. Jonny decided to follow the American dream by starting his own business, JVD Industries, a janitorial service. Despite Gammage's hard work and long hours, the business struggled and eventually failed. In 1990 he was employed as a case-worker for a New York consortium of social services that helped low-income families.

But Seals convinced his cousin in 1992 to move to Tampa Bay to be with him while he played with the Buccaneers. Seals needed a personal manager, someone to take care of everything from maintaining Seals's schedule to making sure his bags were packed on time. Seals, at a time when fame and big money were starting to pour in, wanted someone around him all the time, someone he could trust. He chose his lifelong friend, Jonny Gammage.

When Seals became a free agent in 1994, he signed a major contract with the Steelers and moved to Pittsburgh. Gammage moved with him. Together, they started a business called Athletic Promotions, Inc., which produced and distributed sports T-shirts and other athletic wear featuring the inscription "60 Minute Men," a moniker for the Steelers defense led by Seals. The two men decided that a significant portion of the revenues would go to charitable programs, such as fruit baskets for low-income families and Thanksgiving dinners for those who could not afford their own meals.

"He was more like my brother, my best friend, than my cousin," Seals said. "I am 100 percent committed to seeing that justice is done. I can't bring him back, but I'm concerned with somebody being brought to justice. It's like hanging somebody, how he died. Something is not right here. I know my cousin, and I know he wouldn't jeopardize my job. I know he wouldn't run from the cops. I just want to know what happened."[8] "My cousin would never disrespect you," Seals continued. "The police say he was resisting arrest, but I think he was doing what any normal human being would have done when he's getting hit with a nightstick. He was trying to protect himself."

Gammage's reputation as an upstanding and honorable individual was universal. "It would be very unlike Jonny to have a confrontation with the police," Joseph Citro, a community education activist who had worked with Gammage in Tampa, told the *Post-Gazette*. "He was one of the most peaceable people I know. He was always interested in the community and had begun working for our organization in the local housing development, where he worked with youngsters."9

On Sunday, October 15, I was contacted at home by Robert DelGreco, a prominent and very talented Pittsburgh criminal defense attorney, who had been hired by Ray Seals to investigate his cousin's death. I knew DelGreco mainly through his father, Bobby DelGreco, who had been a childhood friend of mine. In fact, we grew up playing sandlot baseball together. Bobby was so good that he was later signed by the Pittsburgh Pirates to play outfield.

The younger DelGreco asked if I was interested and available to assist in the investigation. At the time, I was not in any governmental position. I had been the Allegheny County coroner for many years, stepping down in the 1980s. But in 1994 several friends and my family had encouraged me to run for the office again. A few months before Gammage's death, I had won the Democratic Party primary.

Because I was facing an opponent in the upcoming general election, I am sure that some of my closest supporters would have wished that I had just watched this case from afar. Everyone knew the case was going to evoke controversy. Everyone knew it pitted black activists against police officers and their supporters. Politically, the potential downside was very significant.

On the other hand, this case provided an example of exactly the situation that I believe that a courageous and honest coroner is expected to face without fear or trepidation. The coroner is an independent authority, sworn to uphold the law. Cases like this, while controversial, can either improve or erode public confidence in our governmental institutions. If the authorities stand up for what is right and just, then the public—white and black—will respect the officers and the office. But if the authorities shy away from pursuing justice just because an issue is controversial or in opposition to public opinion, then the officeholders lose the respect and confidence of the citizenry.

Therefore I never gave a second thought as to whether I should get involved in this case. The Gammage case, I knew, would be one of the most important issues facing Pittsburgh that year. It was my duty to make myself available to help in any way I could.

The Allegheny County coroner's office had conducted the autopsy late on the morning of October 12. DelGreco told me that he would have the coroner's office provide me with an official copy of its autopsy and toxicology reports. But he also asked if I would fly to Syracuse to perform a second autopsy. I agreed.

Wednesday morning, October 18, I took the early morning flight from Pittsburgh to Syracuse. I grabbed my newspapers to read during the flight. The front page of the *Post-Gazette* and the *Tribune-Review* featured articles on the Gammage case, announcing that the Federal Bureau of Investigation was launching its own inquiry into Gammage's death. The articles quoted FBI spokesman Tom Noschese as saying that the agency started its probe as the result of reports about the facts of the case that appeared in the news media.

"Our investigations focus primarily on the level of violence and whether or not it was justified," Noschese stated. "There are a lot of altercations that occur that we would never investigate. In this case here, we had someone who died in connection with a police action. At this point in time, we don't know if there were any violations. But the facts at this time warrant a preliminary investigation."[10]

The FBI officially and publicly announcing that it was conducting an investigation was a major development. It sent the message that the federal government was suspicious of the official police version of the story, and it put the Pittsburgh homicide division on notice that the FBI was looking over its shoulder on this case. This seemed to be a positive development to me. It was also a sign that the US Department of Justice under the Clinton administration had gotten more serious about civil rights violations.

In the same article, acting Allegheny County coroner F. James Gregris announced that he was scheduling a coroner's inquest for November 1, 1995. Under Pennsylvania law, coroners are allowed to conduct inquests that are similar to grand jury inquiries, except that they are open to the public. The purpose of an inquest is to examine whether a death was justified or to see if homicide charges should be brought. The inquests are usually supervised by the coroner, a deputy coroner, or a visiting judge. Usually, a prosecutor from the district attorney's office is asked to question witnesses and present evidence. The coroner's inquest has subpoena power to require testimony, just as a grand jury does. We do not like to subpoena witnesses. We would rather they testify voluntarily. But sometimes witnesses refuse to discuss a matter without a subpoena.

This provision in Pennsylvania law gives the coroner in Pittsburgh the most power or authority of any coroner or medical examiner in the country. Now, 95 percent of the cases involve situations in which the police have already brought charges. In those situations, the inquest is brief and usually closed. But on those rare occasions when a controversy exists over the death and where the police have not charged anyone with the death, the coroner has the authority to conduct the open inquest. These are in cases where the coroner believes that the facts surrounding the death should be aired publicly.

A coroner can also use the open inquest proceedings if he feels that the police or district attorney is failing to conduct a proper investigation of a death. The bottom line is that if the police or the prosecutors do not investigate, and if the coroner doesn't investigate, then nothing is ever done. The truth will never see the light of day.

After reading the newspaper articles on the Gammage case, I opened the envelope that Robert DelGreco, Seals's lawyer, had sent me. It contained two documents: the initial Pittsburgh police report detailing statements made by the officers at the scene of Gammage's traffic stop and the initial Allegheny County coroner's investigative report. They were the first official explanations about what happened the night that Gammage died. However, they were only summary in nature, offering no details and no conclusions. It was the coroner's report on which I focused.

Commonwealth of Pennsylvania

Allegheny County Coroner's Office

Deceased: Gammage, John
Case #: 95-2867
DOB: 07/20/64
Sex: Male
Race: Black
Height: Five feet seven inches
Weight: 187 lbs
Marital Status: Single
Organ Donation: Requested? No   **Permission Given?** No
Official Death: 12 Oct 95 3:51 AM
   At: Mercy Hospital of Pittsburgh
         1400 Locust Street, Pittsburgh, PA
Next of Kin: Johnny & Narves Gammage, Parents

Circumstances of Death:

On 10/12/95 at 1:47 AM, the above male was the driver and lone occupant of a 1988 Jaguar. The above was traveling northbound on S.R. 51 when he committed a moving violation and was told to pull over by Brentwood Police Dept. A pursuit ensued that also included Whitehall P.D. and Baldwin P.D. The above was finally pulled over in the 2100 block of S.R. 51 in front of Duquesne Light Pole 110/004. The above was removed from the vehicle and attempts were made to subdue the above. The above resisted arrest and caused biting injuries to several officers. Once the above was subdued, he went into cardiac arrest at the scene. Brentwood E.M.S. along with Pgh. Medics were dispatched to the scene. Brentwood medics were first to arrive on scene. . . . Resuscitative measures were initiated and the above was transported to Mercy Hospital. Shortly after arrival to Mercy Hospital, the above was pronounced [dead] in the E.R. Dr. Miller (Mercy E.R.) stated that the only noted trauma to the above was an abrasion on the forehead.

Alcohol: No
Drugs: No
Coded Primary Cause of Death: Asphyxiation
Agent: Positional
Mechanism: Strangulation

I also reviewed the toxicology report, which showed that Gammage's urine samples tested by the crime lab were free of any traces of cocaine, marijuana, heroin, PCP, or barbiturates. There were no traces of any drug that would have caused Gammage to behave in an erratic, bizarre, or aggressive manner as described by the police at the scene of his death.

The report showed that Gammage's blood-alcohol level was about 0.04—less than half of the .10 at which someone is legally considered intoxicated or impaired to operate a vehicle. In fact, 0.04 indicates that Gammage may have had one or two beers. Again, the alcohol level revealed nothing that indicated any problem.

Acting Allegheny County coroner James Gregris stated that there was "pressure applied to the neck area and upper chest, which can cut off oxygen and/or the blood supply to the brain, thus leading to death."[11] However, he came to no conclusions as to how or why it happened. He and the coroner's office were obviously leaving those answers up to the coroner's inquest and the jury that would hear it.

Included in the packet were a handful of photographs taken by Pittsburgh police at the scene of the incident on the morning it occurred. The photographs showed Gammage in the middle of the street on his back wearing a dark sweatshirt and jeans. His body lay near the back of the Jaguar on the driver's side.

A member of DelGreco's legal team met me at the Syracuse airport and drove me to the funeral home where Gammage's body lay in state. The funeral was scheduled to start in only a few hours. The funeral home had Gammage's body ready for me to examine. The body had already been embalmed and was prepared for burial. It's always better to conduct an autopsy before the body has been embalmed. As coroners, we do not permit embalming prior to our examination because it causes the organs within the body to change, thus possibly destroying evidence. But in this case the embalming did not in any way compromise my ability to see key elements of the body.

First, I examined the body to see if there was any bruising on the neck, shoulders, or chest. I noted what I believed were about twenty bruises, cuts, or scrapes that could have occurred during the incident, including five internal bruises and hemorrhages on the neck and upper back.

I also looked to see if there was any congestion. Gammage's face was reddish purple. I noticed pinpoint hemorrhages or dots in the lining or whites of the eyes. Severe compression on the chest does not allow the blood to flow from the veins in the head, face, neck, and shoulders back to the heart. Instead, severe compression causes the blood to back up in the smaller veins that lead into the vena cava, which is the large vein draining the blood back to the superior vena cava. The blood from the lower body all the way down to the toes flows back via the inferior vena cava. Both the superior vena cava and the inferior vena cava feed into the first chamber of the heart, the right auricle. In cases of severe compression, the blood becomes backed up and engorged, causing a very prominent discoloration.

In this case, Gammage had no bone fractures. He was a young man, so his bones continued to have a good degree of flexibility. If Gammage had been older, his bones would have been more susceptible to bone fractures from heavy compression.

Finally, I examined the body internally. That's when I noticed that the veins were engorged and there were pinpoint hemorrhages on the surface of the heart. This was more evidence of severe, lengthy compression on the chest. The second autopsy took less than an hour. I thanked the funeral home staff and DelGreco's legal team for having everything ready for me.

Three hours later, more than four hundred people crowded into the funeral home's primary chapel. The memorial service was led by Gammage's pastor, Elder John Lewis of the Full Gospel Church of the Lord. "God, this is another example of what can happen when we think that all is well," Lewis told the congregation. "One of the stars of our universe has fallen."[12]

The Reverend Larry Ellis said Gammage's commitment and love and passion for community service to the underprivileged began when he was only thirteen, when he volunteered to work at a home for senior citizens. "Jonny Gammage was a person who reached out even in high school," Ellis said. "We were robbed of a jewel. Tell Pittsburgh they were robbed. Florida, you were robbed. World, we were robbed."[13]

"Love didn't kill Jonny Gammage," Ellis told the audience. "Hate killed Jonny Gammage."

The next evening, Thursday, October 19, the Reverend Jesse Jackson came to Pittsburgh as part of a program encouraging African American parents to become more closely involved in their children's education. But he used the opportunity to speak out about Jonny Gammage's death.

"Here, there is every evidence that this man was murdered," Jackson stated. "This man was unarmed. He was held down until he could no longer breathe. Those who are guilty must face the full weight of the law. We cannot encourage anyone to engage in any kind of militia. We must operate within the law and the law must be fully enforced. Only when people feel that the law is not enforced do they feel that they do not have equal protection. Then they feel the law is not credible and they attempt to go outside the law and take matters into their own hands. That is why officials must move quickly and move forcefully."[14] "There is not a civil right more basic than the right to live, the right to breathe free," he added.

The Allegheny County coroner's office informed me on Monday, October 24, that it wanted to call me to testify at the open inquest. The coroner's office wanted to know if I would be in Pittsburgh, available, and willing to testify. "Absolutely," I responded.

A few days before the coroner's inquest, I found myself driving north on Route 51, or Saw Mill Run Boulevard—taking the exact route that Jonny Gammage took the night he died. Route 51 leaves Pittsburgh for about 1.4 miles, at which time it is in the town of Brentwood. The communities of Baldwin and Whitehall are literally only a few blocks away, bordering Brentwood to the west and south.

From the police reports I examined, Gammage turned on Route 51, passing a McDonalds and a church. The street is a commercial area, with sports bars, restaurants, retail shops, and service-oriented businesses. There's an Arby's fast-food restaurant, a Michelin Tire store, and the J-Bird restaurant. Route 51 is in a valley between two hills that are speckled with homes. It was fall, with the leaves on the trees turning orange, red, and brown.

I pulled over and got out of my car at the very spot where Gammage stopped for the police—the 2100 block of Route 51—right next to Duquesne Light Pole number 110/004. Directly across the street was Frank & Shirley's restaurant, a family-style diner. As I looked over the scene, I could only imagine what happened during the early morning of October 12. And I wondered if the inquest, which was scheduled to begin just two days later, would produce a full accounting of what had happened, of what went wrong.

At 9 AM on Wednesday, November 1, 1995, the doors to room

313 at the Allegheny County Courthouse opened. More than four hundred people stood in line in the courthouse corridor wanting to witness the inquest. Among them were more than one hundred people—friends and supporters of Gammage's family—who had traveled by bus from Syracuse. But it was clear that not everyone would make it inside.

Most of the 138 seats were actually reserved. Members of the Gammage and Seals families had a row of seats set aside for them. Lawyers and representatives of the five police officers and the police departments involved in the Gammage case were provided chairs. The FBI had two seats. About a dozen seats were reserved for members of the news media. By the time the courtroom was opened to the public, only about fifty seats were available.

Deputy Coroner Arthur G. Gilkes Jr. presided over the inquest. Six jurors—two black women, two white men, one black man, and a white woman—were chosen from the general jury pool to hear the case. Their mission was essentially to decide if the police officers were justified in the amount of force they used against Jonny Gammage. The coroner's jury could decide that the amount of force—and thus Gammage's death—was justified, and that would be the end of it, for all practical purposes. Or the jury could find that the use of force was excessive, that Gammage's death was unjustified, and recommend that homicide charges be brought against one, some, or all of the officers. However, the jury's decision was not binding. It was up to the district attorney to decide whether to officially charge and arrest the officers.

Deputy District Attorney W. Christopher Conrad, who was the lead homicide prosecutor in Allegheny County, handled the case. While the five police officers who were the target of the inquiry and their lawyers were allowed in the inquest to watch, they were not permitted to ask questions. They were told in advance that they could provide written questions to Conrad and he would decide whether or not to ask those questions. The purpose is to keep the inquest as nonadversarial as possible.

Conrad did an expert job of presenting the evidence in chronological order of how things allegedly happened during the early morning hours of October 12. He methodically walked each officer through the specific movements that took place on Route 51.

The first witness was Lt. Milton Mulholland, the Brentwood officer who initially pursued Gammage. The fifty-six-year-old Mulholland was six feet tall, weighed 225 pounds, and had been on the Brentwood police force for twenty-four years. He said he was patrolling the businesses along Route 51 when he first spotted a 1988 Jaguar traveling erratically in the northbound passing lane. The automobile wasn't going fast. Instead, he said the car's brake lights kept coming on every twenty or so feet.

Intrigued and suspicious that the driver might be intoxicated, Mulholland decided to follow the Jaguar. But under oath, he said he could not see if the driver of the car was white or black, man or woman, because the windows were tinted. When he purportedly saw the Jaguar drive through a red light without stopping, he turned on his flashing lights. Mulholland said that the Jaguar did not stop, nor did it speed up. But he said he thought that the vehicle ran through two more traffic lights without stopping. During this so-called slow-speed chase, Mulholland radioed his police dispatcher seeking possible backup and calling in the license tag on the Jaguar.

The police lieutenant testified that Gammage eventually pulled over in the 2100 block of Route 51, next to Frank & Shirley's restaurant, which is just inside the Pittsburgh city limits. The officer said that as soon as the Jaguar stopped, the driver jumped out of the car. Mulholland said he yelled out to the driver to "stay in your car," but the driver continued to walk toward the police cruiser.

Upon repeating the demand, the officer testified that the driver returned to his car and sat down inside with his car door open. Mulholland said that Gammage provided him with his license. But he said Gammage informed the officer that he did not have the vehicle's registration information because the Jaguar actually belonged to his cousin.

It was at about this time that two additional police officers, Patrolman John Vojtas of Brentwood and Sgt. Keith Henderson of Whitehall, arrived at the scene in separate squad cars. Henderson was thirty-six years old, five feet ten inches tall, and weighed 185 pounds. He had been an officer for thirteen years. Vojtas had been a policeman for fifteen years.

Mulholland said he returned to his police cruiser to get the radio dispatcher to run Gammage's name and license number through an Internet-based law enforcement program that keeps track of warrants and criminal records. The dispatcher informed the lieutenant that the computer showed Gammage had no prior criminal record and that there were no warrants for him.

As Mulholland was receiving the information on his police radio, he overheard Officer Henderson tell Gammage to "sit still and quit moving around."

Henderson testified that Gammage was fumbling around for something inside the car. He thought it might be a gun. Instead, Gammage produced what appeared to be a white business card and tried to hand it to one of the officers. Henderson stated that Gammage again reached back inside his car for something and had something else in his hand.

"I noticed as I walked past him that he was making eye contact with me, and at the same time, he was reaching with his right hand between the console and the right side of the driver's seat," Vojtas told the jury. "I asked him, 'Is this your car?' He said, 'Yeah, uh, no.' He was stuttering and acting nervous. I said, 'Well, which is it?' He said, 'It's Mr. Seals's car.' I said, 'I'm sorry, I don't know who Mr. Seals is.' He said, 'He's my cousin and he's a Pittsburgh Steeler.'

"I said, 'Does Mr. Seals know you have this car?'" Vojtas testified. "He said, 'Yeah . . . no . . . yeah.' He was stuttering and acting in a nervous fashion. That was making me nervous."

Vojtas said Gammage kept reaching for something under the console. "I said, 'I'm nervous just like you.' He reached again. I said, 'Hey look, you have to stop reaching,'" Vojtas told the packed courtroom. "I told him, 'That's it. I told you to keep your hands where I can see them. You're scaring me. You're making me nervous.' I felt in an alerted state because he kept refusing my commands."

Vojtas said he finally ordered Gammage to exit the car. "I said, 'Don't come out with anything in your hands.' As he's coming out, his right hand is still between the right side of the seat and the console. His left hand grabbed a date book and what I later found out was a cellular phone," Vojtas testified. "From an alerted state, I became alarmed and drew my weapon," he said. "As I pulled my weapon out, I ordered him to halt. I said, 'Stop! Freeze! Don't even come out of the car,' and he continues to come out of the car. I'm still scared. I don't see his right hand. I start to back up. I start to retreat.

"The driver now rushes toward me," Vojtas stated. "He continues forward and reaches me, and we're chest to chest. I took my forearms and pushed him back to the vehicle. I said, 'Don't move! Freeze! Drop what you have in your hand!' But without any delay, the driver again rushes at me a second time."

Officer Henderson told the jury: "I thought I saw something in his hand. I drew my gun." Henderson said he saw Vojtas knock something from Gammage's hand.

"He rips the flashlight out of my hand and starts swinging it about," Vojtas testified.

Mulholland testified that he went toward Gammage to get the flashlight away from him. "I was struck in the side of the face," the lieutenant told the jury.

"I took the flashlight and hit him several times on the legs," Henderson later testified. "The flashlight had no effect on him. It was a pretty violent struggle."

Mulholland told the jury that Gammage was kicking, punching, and elbowing the officers. "Mr. Gammage continued to struggle," he said. "Eventually we collapsed to the pavement. I was under Gammage."

Mulholland said that the other two officers, Henderson and Vojtas, grabbed Gammage's arms and were trying to apply handcuffs when Gammage started to get back up. They knocked Gammage back to the pavement, this time on his stomach. By this time, Whitehall officer Shawn Patterson and Baldwin Borough officer Michael Albert had arrived. Mulholland stated that he saw Patterson on Gammage's back, hitting the suspect on the legs with his flashlight, while Albert was sitting on Gammage's back, holding him down with a baton.

Mulholland, who had undergone heart bypass surgery a few years earlier, testified that the brief but intense struggle had left him "physically spent, close to exhaustion." He told the jury that he crawled away from the fight for a few minutes.

Vojtas said that in order to get better control, he placed his knee on Gammage's back because the suspect was acting so violently. The officer testified that while his arms were around Gammage from behind trying to put the handcuffs on, Gammage bit him. "He clamped down on my right thumb," Vojtas stated. "His fighting behavior is still continuing but now he's biting down on my thumb. I'm thinking, he's going to bite my thumb off."

Vojtas said he punched Gammage four or five times on the jaw to get Gammage to stop biting. "It didn't seem to faze him," Vojtas testified. "He kept clamping down harder and harder. I was in shock, starting to black out, and before I knew it, I was able to get my thumb free." Vojtas said he withdrew from the fight to make sure his thumb was okay and then returned to help finish the handcuffing.

"I was upset," Vojtas stated. "I looked at my thumb. It was swollen three times its normal size. The AIDS thing went through my mind. I said, 'I hope you don't have AIDS, because if I'm going to die, I hope you die.' I had no idea he was in serious condition."

Officer Albert, who had been on the Baldwin police force for three years and had been a military police officer for seven years, said that "a violent fight on the ground" was underway when he arrived.

"I approached Gammage from the rear," Albert told the jury. "He's facedown and I attempted to put pressure on his upper back with my hands to hold him down. There was a lot of thrashing around. Vojtas said he was getting bitten. He was screaming in pain. I stood up and got my collapsible baton. I crouched over Mr. Gammage once again, grabbed either end of the baton, and tried to apply pressure across the shoulders. Vojtas raised his hand and I saw it was blood-covered. It was less than thirty seconds. I used the force I thought could meet the resistance of him trying to raise upwards."

Albert stated that Gammage knocked the baton away. Vojtas then instructed Albert to place his foot on Gammage's neck.

"I applied pressure to hold Mr. Gammage on the ground," Albert said. "I didn't want my hands anywhere near him after I saw what he did to Officer Vojtas. I had my foot on his neck a very short time because, with all the thrashing about, I couldn't really put pressure because I lost my balance. It was maybe ten seconds. I knelt down on my right knee on the ground and my left knee on his back, once again for a very short time, less than probably twenty seconds."

The fifth officer to testify was Whitehall patrolman Shawn Patterson, the last of the police officers to be involved with Gammage the morning of October 12. Patterson, a nine-year police veteran, said he decided to go to the scene only when he heard the police dispatcher repeatedly trying to reach officers already at the scene but getting no radio response. The thirty-one-year-old suburban officer told the jury that he arrived at the scene of a "violent melee going on." He testified that Gammage was lying facedown when he arrived and that Officers Henderson and Vojtas were on his upper body and Lieutenant Mulholland was on his legs.

"Mr. Gammage just wouldn't listen," Patterson stated. "They were telling him, 'Just be still. You're under arrest.' Everyone was screaming orders but Gammage was responding violently, trying to strike all of the officers."

Patterson said that Lieutenant Mulholland's face "was beet red. It was going through my mind that Lieutenant Mulholland was going to die. I knew about his heart problems." Patterson testified that he struck Gammage several times with his blackjack, believing that would help immobilize him.

Vojtas told the coroner's jury that he radioed for an ambulance to treat him for his bleeding thumb. He also told the dispatcher that the operator of the vehicle might also need medical attention. Minutes later, the paramedics arrived and helped apply leg restraints on Gammage.

It was about that moment that Gammage yelled out: "Keith, Keith. I'm 31. I'm only 31."

That's when Matthew Fox, one of the Brentwood paramedics on the scene, testified that he heard "a popping noise" and a "sharp inward breath" come from Gammage's body. Fox told the jury that two officers were kneeling on Gammage's shoulders at the time.

It was then that Officer Henderson noticed that Gammage was no longer struggling. In fact, he was not moving at all.

"I said, 'Get off him!' At which time they all did," Fox testified. The paramedics had the officers turn Gammage onto his back. There was no pulse. They immediately started cardiopulmonary resuscitation, also known as CPR. They also used a defibrillator on Gammage several times.

"Still, they got no heartbeat," Patterson told the jury. "I was very concerned for Mr. Gammage. I thought to myself that I hope they get a heartbeat, but they continued CPR and they didn't."

Gammage was immediately transported to nearby Mercy Hospital, where he was officially pronounced dead at 3:51 AM.

After Gammage had been taken to the hospital, the officers searched his car for illegal drugs or alcohol or a weapon. All they found was a moldy bag of marijuana. And crime lab officials testified that they tested Gammage's blood and found no trace of any illegal substances.

During the three-day hearing, Conrad called thirty-eight witnesses to testify. Ray Seals told the jury that his cousin was a peaceful man who had never been in trouble. A couple of eyewitnesses who drove by the scene the morning of October 12 said they saw the five officers huddled over the motionless body of Gammage, not helping him at all. Other witnesses stated that Gammage's cell phone would not work if it wasn't plugged into the car, so it was unlikely he had it in his hand as the officers testified. Brentwood police chief Babish testified that Lieutenant Mulholland admitted to him immediately after the incident that he had put Gammage in a headlock at the scene—a statement Mulholland denied during his portion of the testimony.

The final two witnesses called by Deputy District Attorney Christopher Conrad to testify were Dr. Abdulrezak Shakir, a deputy medical examiner in the Allegheny County coroner's office, and myself. Each of us walked the jury, the prosecutor, and the audience through our examinations of the body and how Jonny Gammage died. Our analysis and conclusions were essentially the same.

As a forensic pathologist being called as a witness, my main goal is always to explain highly technical information in as simple a manner as possible. I feel it is my mission to educate the jury, to get them to understand what I know. In the Gammage case, I was on the witness stand for only about thirty minutes. Mr. Conrad did an excellent job of walking me and the jury through the key forensic elements of the case.

> **Conrad:** Good afternoon, doctor. Would you state your name for the record, please?
> **Wecht:** Cyril H. Wecht.
> **Conrad:** You are a physician and forensic pathologist?
> **Wecht:** Yes, sir.
> **Conrad:** You are also an attorney?
> **Wecht:** Yes.
> **Conrad:** Doctor, you were brought into this case to review this particular matter by members interested in—the Gammage

family—interested in what had happened to Mr. Gammage; is that fair to say?

Wecht: Yes. I was contacted by attorney Robert DelGreco, who informed me he was representing Mr. Ray Seals and the family of Mr. Gammage.

Conrad: You listened to Dr. Shakir testify immediately prior to you. Are you in agreement with his final opinion to a reasonable degree of medical certainty as to what caused Mr. Gammage's death?

Wecht: Yes, I am in agreement. I would consider this to be a case of mechanical asphyxiation due to compression of the chest.

Conrad: Tell us, why don't you, you can start with a general explanation even of the mechanical asphyxia and continue for us, please.

Wecht: What do I believe, I believe that there was primarily compression of the chest with a significant reduction in Mr. Gammage's ability to have normal respiratory excursion. Just think of it as a compressive force similar to a workman in a ditch, and mud or sand moves in on both sides. His head can be completely above the debris, no obstruction at all to his nose and mouth, but he can't move his chest. In this case, Mr. Gammage's chest in the front was pinned against a hard, unyielding surface, and his back was pinioned by one or more police officers with various parts of their body. So you have then, as Dr. Shakir has discussed, a markedly inhibited ability of the respiratory and abdominal components, the thoracic [the area between the neck and the abdomen that contains the heart and lungs in a bony cage of vertebrae] and abdominal components to participate in normal respiratory excursion, movement of the chest. And the more weight you have, the greater is the compressive force, and the longer the weight is applied, the more physiological problems evolve. I think that I would like to perhaps emphasize something: there is then an evolving degree of hypoxia, which is decreased oxygenation as opposed to anoxia, which means total deprivation of oxygen. As this impediment continues with the chest and pulmonary function, then there is going to be some deprivation of oxygen and that is going to play out with the heart muscle and play out with the brain.

Conrad: For instance with the heart, how is it affecting the heart muscle?

Wecht: It is producing these very minor subtle changes that can insult the heart, irritate the muscle by the myocardial fibers, and cause it to beat erratically or arrhythmically. . . . Dr. Shakir talked about ventricular fibrillation [chaotic contractions across the atrium of the heart]. That is probably the ultimate mechanism. We can't see it at the autopsy table, but more likely than not there was another arrhythmia that preceded ventricular fibrillation. It is not often you will go to ventricular fibrillation unless you have a bunch of heart attacks, a massive heart attack, or so on.

Conrad: There is no indication, of course, of that in Mr. Gammage?

Wecht: No, absolutely not. And I asked about prior medical history to make absolutely certain, and the examination of the heart and microscope reveals a perfectly normal heart you would expect in a thirty-one-year-old male.

Conrad: Could the pressure being applied, could it have a cumulative effect if it is interrupted for a brief period of time and then reinstituted, was . . . this a cumulative effect?

Wecht: I would agree with Dr. Shakir's explanation. If you have somebody who is unable to breathe and who is struggling for air—which is the most fundamental primitive physiological reflex in the part of any living entity, any animal in the animal kingdom, not just human beings—if you then remove that pressure and oxygen gets in, then you will have complete restoration in a relatively short period of time of the state of respiratory normalcy. It is possible, if the pressure had been applied for some time, you could have had some focal areas of damage to the brain or to the heart. These would be microscopic, quite subtle. They could be more severe if it had gone on, but like people who go into cardiac arrest and they may be salvaged [within] four or five minutes, [but] six minutes later and [they] have permanent brain damage, and you can have a persistent vegetative state, they are not quite as sharp, but in the situation involving some seconds or a minute or so it is all going to come back. You can still have a little lingering effect in the heart muscle fibers and in the brain. So that if the compressive force is reapplied subsequently, you have a more susceptible physiological state, and I think it would be easier then for these problems to evolve than if it had just been started initially without any prior insult.

Conrad: Can you offer us any opinion from your experience and your study of this particular case, clinical study of this particular case, of how long this force would have needed to have been applied and what amount of force needed to be applied or could have been responsible?

Wecht: With regard to the amount of force, I would say that the amount of force had to be substantial. In a thirty-one-year-old healthy male with a good body musculature, which Mr. Gammage had, and with significant flexibility of the bony thorax [the bony area in the chest that protects the lungs and heart], there is still a lot of cartilage there, it is not all hard bone like it comes to be in those of us who grow older, you have much resiliency. In order to compress the chest to the point that it is compromising the ability to breathe, you have to have substantial force, and in this case, I think what we are talking about is weight, weight directly from one or more people, weight applied indirectly through the use of some instrumentality, what has been referred to possibly as a baton or so on. So the force must be substantial. With regards to the length of time of this application, I think it has to be sustained over a period of a few minutes. I do not believe that the transient application of force or that the application of substantial force that isn't breaking anything inside, that isn't producing any hemorrhage, that isn't tearing any internal organs, that is just causing problems by virtue of the pressure, that you are not going to reach a point of dying in a matter of seconds or a couple of minutes because the fact is, you and I drop right now for whatever reason and if they can get to us with good oxygen and good CPR technique, in four minutes we are probably going to recover with no brain damage at all and may go [as long as] five or six minutes.

The Court: Doctor, it would be your opinion that this force lasted for in excess of five minutes?

Wecht: I believe so, Your Honor, because this was not an anoxic state, this was not total deprivation of oxygen, this was diminished ability to obtain oxygen. So hypoxia [loss of blood supply and inadequate oxygenation] takes longer. When I just talked to Mr. Conrad a moment ago about that four-minute collapse and so on, I am talking about no oxygen. Now, if you have just decreased oxygen, then lengthen the period of time.

Conrad: So it is your opinion he wasn't just entirely deprived of oxygen from the time . . . prior to his death but. . . .

Wecht: No, I don't believe he was totally deprived of oxygen. That would be very hard to do because if you are going to have that kind of force, you are probably going to get some fractures. You can only . . . you can get some resiliency as I talked, but in order to cut things off and stop all ability to breathe, you are going to have to have a great amount of force, and I think you would have: A, fractures, and B, more internal damage to soft tissues and organs in the neck and even possibly the apices, the upper portions of the lungs.

Conrad: I will ask this question. If Mr. Gammage had the breath knocked out of him, so to speak, in his initial fall, would that particular state indicate to you that it would take less time for this mechanism to have had the effect that it had on him?

Wecht: Well, that is a phrase that we have all used in a colloquial sense. It is difficult for me medically to understand what it means to define [what] it was to have the breath knocked out of you literally. It could be a spontaneous pneumothorax in which air escapes from the lungs and you change, and the pressure gradients in the chest cavity, but I don't think that is what anybody is talking about and certainly is not applicable here. If you have somebody who had the breath knocked out of them for some reason and you immediately begin to compress the chest, the answer is obvious, it is going to kick in faster than it would otherwise. But if on the other hand the person has the breath knocked out of him and then starts to breathe normally, then everything is back to square one, and you have to then begin the compromising force application at that time.

Conrad: One of the paramedics indicated he heard a popping sound immediately prior to him being diagnosed as arresting. Do you have any opinion what that could have been?

Wecht: I think it was a respiratory sound, probably a forcible expulsion of air. It certainly was not related to any kind of disruption of the musculoskeletal system, no fracture or dislocation.

Conrad: You obviously limited all the natural . . . eliminated all the natural causes of death?

Wecht: Yes. I think it can be stated quite unequivocally and unhesitatingly there are no natural disease processes of any kind which could have even remotely contributed in any way either to any alleged or perceived behavioral problem or to any pathological process that would have set the stage for his death or which would have caused his death.

Conrad: Obviously, there is an indication that Officer Vojtes was bitten by Mr. Gammage here and quite severely. Could you, knowing the clinical history of what was going on there, can you offer an explanation for what state Mr. Gammage might have been in when that occurred?

Wecht: Well, I have already said, and all of us know, and I hope this is not considered to be a sexist remark, but most women don't play football. We all know from football and the kind of wild things as little boys, Buck Buck, King of the Hill, everybody piles on, and knows what it is like not to be able to breathe. It is the most horrible feeling in the world, and you are going to struggle and it is going to [be] voluntary and conscious. And as Dr. Shakir talked about, if you are moving into a state of semidelirium and so on, involuntary reflexes are going to kick in immediately and you are going to be trying very hard to breathe. That is one observation I would make. Another one, I don't know how much it is in the realm of forensic pathology, but maybe a little bit based on experience from that aspect that when an adult man gets into a fight with another adult man, biting is not usually part of the weaponry that is employed. The biting to me, you know, is strongly suggestive of a struggle to get the mouth or the head free so that the person can breathe.

Conrad: Dr. Shakir testified in one of the three mechanisms of death based upon trauma, in the areas of trauma to which he spoke, one did involve reflex, basically reflex action?

Wecht: Vagal reflex, that is correct. That certainly could have played a part here, because the vagus nerve [which runs from the throat to the abdominal area] has a subduing effect on the heart and when it is excited or irritated, it will cause the heart to be even slower, bradycardia, and that can set ventricular fibrillation, which is the worse kind of arrhythmia because while the heart moves, no blood is pumped out. Ventricular fibrillation, think of a shivering snake, it wiggles and no blood is pumped.

Conrad: In your opinion, as this is happening to Mr. Gammage in the company of the police officers, what indication are they going to have watching him that this, that this process is going to an eventually unalterable state or inalterable state?

Wecht: Well, it is difficult to answer without engaging in too much conjecture, and with a desire to be reasonable about this, I cannot attribute medical knowledge to police officers pertaining to these kind of pathophysiological processes that we talked about and so on. However, I do believe that police officers in modern times, those who have been around for a couple of years, have a pretty good idea of how people react when they feel that they are having difficulty in breathing, and I do believe in the year 1995 that police officers in America should be very much aware of the fact that somebody who is in a prone position, lying on their abdomen, is much more susceptible to respiratory compromise than other people. And I do believe that police officers are aware that when somebody is struggling in that kind of a position that once you get handcuffs on, then you take them out of the prone position. Whether you leave them supine, sit them up, or stand them up—that is your decision based on what is available—but you don't leave them in a prone position and you do not continue to apply force and pressure to the back as they are struggling. The last thing in the world you want to do is to continue to say, okay, man, you keep struggling and I am going to keep applying more force to your back and so on. What is the end result? What are you, in fact, saying? I am going to keep doing this until you are not struggling. Well, you will not be struggling if you are not breathing.

The coroner's jury deliberated about seventy minutes before returning to the courtroom with its decision. The five white police officers should be arrested and charged with homicide, the panel concluded unanimously. None of the five officers were in the courtroom when the verdict was announced.

Shouts of "Hallelujah!" and "Praise the Lord!" were heard throughout the courtroom and in the hallways of the court house. Some people in the courtroom cried while others raised their hands heavenward in prayer. "That's what was served today—pure justice," one spectator told news reporters. Ray Seals sat quietly in the front row, hugged family members, and shook hands with others.

"We felt the police officers lied in trying to cover it up—all five of them," juror Beth Beeler, a thirty-four-year-old hospice nurse, told the *Post-Gazette* following the announcement of the verdict.

"They were insulting our intelligence. We felt they knew something more that wasn't forthcoming, and we felt we needed to send a strong message this type of behavior would not be tolerated. We really felt this was done because he was a black male."[15]

Following the verdict, Deputy Coroner Arthur Gilkes, who presided over the inquest, publicly announced that he agreed with the jury's findings and that he would recommend to the Allegheny County district attorney, Bob Colville, that charges be brought against the officers. "This was a traffic stop on one of the streets of our county," Gilkes said. "Definitely citizens should not expect to wind up in a cemetery for a routine traffic stop."[16]

A few weeks after the coroner's inquest, prosecutors officially brought charges against three of the five officers. But problems immediately arose with the cases. First, Mr. Conrad was replaced as lead prosecutor. Second, new prosecutors decided to try the three officers separately. Why does this matter? In my opinion, it was strategically important to try all five officers together to show how their combined actions caused the death of Jonny Gammage. The asphyxiation resulted from the individual actions of all the officers working together. One officer pressed on Gammage's upper back. Another was pressuring his buttocks. Another was putting his weight against the shoulders. Someone else had a foot against the back of his neck. By agreeing to separate their cases at trial, the defense attorneys for the officers were able to argue very effectively that the individual actions of their clients pressuring Gammage at this spot for this amount of time could not have caused his death. And by trying the officers separately, it became more difficult to show what each officer's role was and what each officer did exactly to Gammage that morning.

Consequently, the cases ended in mistrials, and no convictions were ever obtained. The Gammage family sued the police departments for wrongful death and civil rights violations—lawsuits that ended up being settled out of court for an undisclosed amount of money.

In addition, the US Department of Justice, after a lengthy investigation, chose not to prosecute the officers. Federal prosecutors were sympathetic to the Gammage family but concluded that they simply would not win their case at trial. Police brutality and civil rights cases are tough to win because juries want to believe police officers. There's a general sympathy toward police officers for what a tough job they have and how they are protecting us. In addition, in most of these cases, the police officers are white and the victims are black or Latino, which shouldn't make a difference, but any honest lawyer or jury expert will tell you that unfortunately it still does.

That being said, just because the cases are tough to win, that doesn't mean the cases shouldn't be brought. Sometimes you prosecute a case because it is simply the right thing to do. Another reason, I believe, that the Gammage case was never fully prosecuted was that this case was a political hot potato for the administration. Pressure on the federal government to prosecute died down after the family settled its civil lawsuit. The family could fight for only so long.

What do I think happened?

We will never know for sure, of course. Let me say this: I do not believe there was intent to kill Jonny Gammage on the part of the police officers. I find no evidence to indicate that there was any premeditation to kill him. But I do think the officers decided they were going to teach him a lesson. Maybe Gammage did give Vojtas a dirty look. Maybe he did exchange words with the officers. Maybe he did act arrogantly or mouth off. But think about it. Here's a young black man driving a Jaguar through an all-white part of town doing nothing wrong. He wasn't speeding. He wasn't dealing drugs. He wasn't intoxicated. He was merely driving slowly late at night, braking often as if he were searching for an address. Then he gets pulled over by a white police officer, who minutes later is joined by four more white police officers—all on the heels of the Rodney King beating case in Los Angeles. Gammage was an intelligent guy. He had done nothing wrong. He probably felt he was being targeted by white police officers just because of the color of his skin. He probably felt he was entitled to some respect. The officers probably thought Gammage was being smart-alecky. And things then escalated out of control.

It can be very disquieting to someone who feels he has done nothing wrong to be treated in an unfriendly, disrespectful manner. But too frequently, that's the way some officers act.

Did he fight back during the efforts to arrest him? Absolutely. You and I would have done the very same thing if we had been in those same circumstances. Do you want to know why? Because it is psychologically and physiologically automatic for our bodies to react that way when our lives are in danger. Jonny Gammage was struggling because he couldn't breathe. The struggle was interpreted as resistance.

Such a big deal was made that he bit the officer. Well, what did the officers expect? If you put your hand over the mouth and nose of the most obedient, friendly, peaceful dog—your lifetime friend and pet—and cut off his oxygen flow, see how long it is before he bites you. Gammage wasn't biting because he thought he could escape. He certainly wasn't thinking he could bite his way out of the situation. Think about it reasonably. It was a totally defensive reaction. He bit because he couldn't breathe.

The weight of the officers pressing on Gammage's back meant he couldn't breathe because the respiratory muscles, especially the diaphragm, which is the principal muscle involved in respiration, were compressed. The diaphragm is a big tentlike muscle that separates the chest from the abdomen, beneath the lungs, and is protected by the rib cage. When it cannot move freely in an unrestricted fashion, the lungs cannot open and close, and move up and down in a normal manner. Breathing is then compromised. Oxygenation is diminished. The heart and brain are denied oxygen.

It's not that everyone would die under these circumstances or even that Jonny Gammage would have died under these identical circumstances on another day. Complicating the situation was the fact that Gammage was probably excited by the confrontation with the police, causing his metabolism to increase, thus increasing the demand for oxygen. That aggravated the situation.

Then there's the issue of whether the officers should have noticed that Gammage couldn't breathe or was dying. I recognize that the officers are not medical experts. Even so, they should be trained to recognize certain medical conditions. In this case, Gammage essentially told the officers he was in trouble when he spoke his final words: "I'm 31. I'm only 31." What reasonable inference can be made of that statement? Well, to me, there is only one reasonable inference from that statement. He wasn't telling them it was his birthday or inviting them to a party. He wasn't letting them know that he was older or younger than he looked. He said it because he was afraid for his life. He said that because he felt that he was dying.

We will never know what really happened during the early morning hours of October 12 because the police officers all stuck together. Over the past twenty or thirty years, we have seen the wall of silence within the medical and legal professions fall. There used to be a time when doctors would never turn on one of their own, even if they strongly believed their fellow physician was engaged in medical malpractice. The same was true with lawyers. But that is no longer the situation. Doctors and lawyers are eager to police their ranks. They are quick to call the appropriate authorities if they witness one of their own committing a serious error or a crime. They do not hesitate to testify against a professional brother if the brother has gone awry.

That simply is not the case in law enforcement. Despite all the negative cases of police brutality and abuse, officers seem to have more of a circle-the-wagons mentality than ever before. The blue code of silence is just as bad, maybe even worse, than it has ever been.

Having said all that, I need to say this, too: being a police officer is a very tough job. Officers are extremely underpaid. Their salaries should be significantly increased—maybe doubled. If I were to run for mayor of a city, I would campaign on two issues: increasing pay of public school teachers and increasing the pay and training of police officers. I would work with the police unions and police leadership to develop additional training programs that would increase salaries to attract better-qualified candidates. College degrees in criminal justice would be preferred, if not mandated. Psychological testing and evaluation would be conducted for all new officers and redone annually. It's shameful that this has not happened.

Everything about this case was a tragedy. There was simply no reason for this death to have occurred. It's equally as shameful that the cases were not fully prosecuted. The good news is that there's no statute of limitations on murder. The cases can still be reopened. With diligent police work and pressure on the officers to be truthful about what happened, I still feel that justice can be achieved in the death of Jonny Gammage. But time is running out.

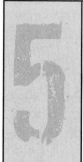

THE CAPTAIN'S DEATH

SUICIDE, MURDER, OR ACCIDENT?

To Lucy Garcia, Jeffrey Digman seemed like the ideal guy. He was handsome, physically fit, and much more mature than the other guys she had dated. At age thirty, Jeffrey sported a military-style buzz cut and a dazzling smile. She thought he drank a little too much at times and could be a little uptight or intense, but he was a good guy and treated her like a princess.

Lucy's alarm clock sounded early the morning of Monday, January 23, 1989. She arose earlier than normal because Jeffrey was coming home and she had a lot to do. She had met US Marine Corp Capt. Jeffrey Digman only a few months earlier, not long after he began his stint in Puerto Rico, where Lucy lived.

Jeffrey had called Lucy a few days earlier from his home in Temecula, California, letting her know he would be returning home that next Monday. He gave her his flight information and itinerary. Jeffrey was meticulous about being prompt and hated waiting. She needed to be there early, waiting for him to land.

He also asked her to take his dress blue uniform and a shirt to the dry cleaners and to have it ready for him when he got back. Jeffrey told her he had an extremely important function to attend that Monday so he needed to look his best. "He told me to inspect it carefully and that if there is even one wrinkle, to take it back and make them fix it," Lucy later said. "He made a very big deal out of how important it was that the uniform be absolutely perfect."[1]

Lucy dressed that Monday morning in one of Jeffrey's favorite outfits. She picked up his uniform at the cleaners and headed to the airport. She was there plenty early, well before his flight arrived. She stood at the gate, almost giddy at the thought of seeing him again, even though they had been apart for only two weeks.

One by one, people on the flight from Atlanta to San Juan stepped off the plane. There were those in first class. And then more streamed by. But no Jeffrey. The last few passengers straggled off about a minute apart from each other. She wondered if he was helping someone else get their bags or possibly, knowing Jeffrey, flirting with a flight attendant.

Finally, the pilots and flight attendants emerged. There was no one else on the plane. In tears, Lucy went to the airline ticket counter, asking if Jeffrey Digman had been moved to another flight. The airline said he had not, but that he hadn't made any of his flights that day.

Back in Southern California, Jeffrey's parents, Bill and Donna Digman, were at home on Sunday evening, January 22, watching television. The telephone rang. Bill answered.

"I've got some very bad news," the caller stated. "Jeffrey is dead. He committed suicide."[2]

The couple couldn't believe it. They didn't believe it. Each of them had talked to Jeffrey just days earlier. True, he seemed a bit depressed and upset. But not suicidal. Not suicidal by a long stretch. But the caller, who was Jeffrey's housemate and also a military officer, said that they should come by right away. They jumped into their 280ZX and drove immediately to their son's home, which was about a half hour away.

The Digmans were met at the front door by their son's roommate, Maj. Douglas K. Wood, who informed them that the coroner was inside conducting an investigation and that the house itself was off-limits to everyone other than law enforcement.

"Did Jeffrey leave a note?" Bill asked.[3]

The major, who lived at and co-owned the home at 39651 June Court in Temecula with Captain Digman, said he had not.

"Then it wasn't suicide," Bill responded. "If it had been a suicide, I am certain Jeffrey would have left a note."[4]

When Bill asked his son's roommate if he had any idea why Jeffrey would take his own life, Major Wood stated, "He didn't want to go back to Puerto Rico."[5]

The major proceeded to tell the Digmans that he and his girlfriend had just returned from a weekend in Las Vegas. He said that when he pulled into the driveway and saw lights on inside the house and found the garage door unlocked, he knew something was wrong. Inside the modest, two-story, tan stucco home, Major Wood said he found the body of Jeffrey Digman lying on his bed in the master bedroom upstairs.

Three days later, on Wednesday, January 25, the Riverside County coroner's office issued its findings in a twelve-page report.

Name: Jeffrey Scott Digman
Sex: Male
Age: 30
DOB: 06/06/1958
Place of Birth: Anaheim, CA
Height: Six feet seven inches
Weight: 154 lbs
Race: Caucasian
Hair: Brown
Eyes: Hazel
Summary of Case: 30 year Marine Officer found by roommate about 2205 [hours or 10:05 PM] lying fully dressed, except for shoes and socks, across his bed with a gunshot wound apparent to the right temporal area behind the ear and an exit wound to the left rear of his head. A .44 Magnum

revolver was found lying between his legs with one expended round behind the hammer. A small abrasion was observed on his right upper cheek. No other trauma was noted to his body and no signs of foul play [were] observed. The body was cold to the touch and in full rigor mortis with lividity consistant [sic] with the position of the body. The ambient temperature of the room at 0051 [or 12:51 AM] was 70 degrees. His liver temperature at 0055 [or 12:55 AM] was recorded at 91 degrees.

Details: Victim was lying in the bed sideways with his face up looking towards the ceiling. Digman's arms were at his side with his feet hanging off the side of the bed. Digman was wearing a blue short-sleeve shirt, faded black jeans, no shoes, no socks, and a black Timex watch. Digman had a hole on the right side of face and a hole on the left side of face behind his ear [this appears to be the bullet's exit point]. Digman was lying on his back in his own blood. Their [sic] was a gun on the floor between Digman's legs. Blood was splattered on the south bedroom wall over the sliding glass door with a hole near the top of the wall [possible bullet exit]. Their [sic] was a brown paper bag containing five empty Budweiser bottles of beer on the floor near the wooden desk.

Cause of Death: Gunshot wound to the head.

Under the category "Classification of Death," there were five choices: Natural, Traffic, Homicide, Suicide, and Accident. The box next to "Suicide" had an "x" typed in it.

As part of the report, officials with the Riverside coroner also included in their written report that they spoke with Major Wood the night the body was discovered.

"Wood stated that Digman was home on leave and was very depressed. Wood stated that Digman was a loner, had no social life, and a very uptight and intense person," according to the report. "Wood said Digman was a heavy drinker and would drink and stay shut up in his room and talk to him. Wood stated Digman, himself, and [his girlfriend] were watching *Full Metal Jacket* on Tuesday (01/17/89) around 8 PM and he became very upset and disturbed about the movie."[6] [The movie depicts a Marine corporal who cannot handle the stress and pressure of military life and shoots himself in the head.]

The report by the Riverside coroner's office seemed somewhat sloppily put together. There were numerous misspellings and poor use of grammar. Every conclusion and analysis stated in the report pointed to suicide.

For their part, military investigators interviewed several of Jeffrey Digman's Marine colleagues, friends, and family. A portion of the picture they painted was of a very emotionally and psychologically disturbed young man who took his own life. While some of his family and other friends, including his girlfriend, agreed that Jeffrey was a bit depressed and even moody, they did not believe he was close to being suicidal.

On February 1, 1989, the Department of the Navy, which conducted the military investigation, released its own findings called a "Report of Casualty." The one-page document noted such diverse facts as Captain Digman's monthly salary was $2,538.90 and he was a Presbyterian by faith. It noted that his "Duty Status" was "active—on authorized leave." The bottom line in the navy's report was that the military believed that the "cause and circumstances" of Captain Digman's death was a "self-inflicted gunshot wound to the head."

Suicide.

Case closed.

Wearing the military blue uniform that Lucy had dry-cleaned, Jeffrey Digman was buried on January 30 with full military honors at the Riverside National Cemetery in California.

Captain Digman wasn't a famous celebrity, so his death received no media attention. Newspapers and television rarely publicize suicides unless the person is well known or unless the suicide itself is something bizarre or spectacular, such as jumping out the window of a skyscraper during rush-hour traffic. Suicides are human tragedies that seldom if ever get wide attention. This case was viewed as simply someone who just couldn't go on living anymore.

About eight months later, in the middle of October 1989, I received a call from Ted L. Gunderson, a private investigator who was working with the Digman family. Ted was no ordinary private eye. He was a former FBI agent who had been the head of the bureau's office in Los Angeles. He was highly respected by prosecutors and law enforcement authorities for being honest and straightforward.

My telephone conversation with Ted was brief but to the point. Digman's parents had hired him to look into their son's death because they didn't believe he killed himself. Ted told me that, after a preliminary investigation, he also had doubts. Strong doubts.

"The investigation by the military and the local authorities was a complete joke," he told me. "Absolutely ridiculous."

Ted said that the goal was to convince the authorities—civilian and military—to reopen the investigation to get to the truth. He said the military had agreed to reexamine the medical evidence in Jeffrey's death, including the possibility of exhuming Jeffrey's body and conducting a second autopsy. If that happened, he told me, they would want our own forensic pathologist to be present at the new autopsy.

"Are you interested and are you available?" Ted asked.

"I'm very interested. It sounds like a fascinating case," I told him. "But you must know, I'm not going to shade my opinion. If I think he committed suicide, that's what I'm going to say."

Ted told me he expected nothing less.

A few days later, on October 27, I received a letter in the mail from Bill Digman, Jeffrey's father. With the brief letter was a packet of information regarding his son's death.

"I am taking the liberty of sending you this collection of data relating to our son," he wrote. "Jeffrey died under suspicious circumstances by a gunshot wound to his head. Our immediate task is to determine beyond doubt whether his death was a suicide or homicide. We are in need of your services to attend and possibly assist in a second autopsy that is to be conducted by the Naval Investigative Services (NIS) pathologist in the near future."

Included in the packet were a series of documents related to Captain Digman and his death:

(1) The original autopsy report and official investigative findings.

(2) A two-page bio about Jeffrey prepared by Mr. Digman. It told how Jeffrey loved to exercise, running about ten miles daily and working out by using weights. He received his bachelor's of science degree in aeronautical engineering from San Jose State University before joining the US Marine Corp. He had been an executive officer in Korea and the Philippines and had been a series commander over recruiting in San Diego.

(3) A six-page letter, dated August 8, from Bill Digman to the Riverside coroner's office in which he detailed his reasons for seeking a reopening of the investigation into their son's death. The letter listed twenty-seven points of controversy or unanswered questions. The letter concluded with Mr. Digman's heartfelt disappointment: "The absence of a military investigation of Jeffrey's death, as required by their own regulations, appears to us that our son was just disposed of like a worn-out shoe."

While many of Mr. Digman's points or issues were those of a concerned father and had little relevance to the manner of death, one thing did stand out: Jeffrey had allegedly shot himself on the right side of his head in the temporal area. However, Jeffrey was left-handed. Just being left-handed doesn't mean he could not have shot himself with his right hand. But it would have been atypical of suicides. As a matter of statistics, people who commit suicide by shooting themselves almost always use their favored or strongest hand. It's probably because that hand and arm are stronger and steadier, and it takes some strength to pull the trigger.

Again, this point did not rule out suicide by any means. But it did raise a question in my mind.

(4) Jeffrey's official Marine fitness report, completed in 1988, was also in the packet. The report said that Captain Digman possessed "unimpeachable personal integrity, a thirst for excellence" and was the "best in his command." The review said that he was "dedicated, hardworking, extremely conscientious, honest and thorough." The report, which was part of Captain Digman's review, stated that he was a "responsible and committed professional," had a "selfless devotion to duty," and "possesses the highest integrity and courage of his convictions."

(5) Finally, there was a thirty-page document prepared by Donna Digman, Jeffrey's mother, regarding the last few days of her son's life. It detailed her conversations with Jeffrey, as well as conversations she had with Major Wood, Lucy Garcia, and others. I can only imagine the pain and tears that went into preparing such a document—having to relive it all.

As I read the document, I found Mrs. Digman to be heartbroken, wondering what she could have done and what others could have done to save her son's life. She was brutally honest in her assessment, discussing Jeffrey's troubled mental state, but also sowing seeds of doubt about whether he could or would commit suicide. The same document had also been presented to the officials at the Riverside coroner's office.

Before I go on, let me state this upfront: in cases of suicide, it is very common for family members and close friends to refuse to believe that the person they loved would actually end his or her own life, especially in a violent manner. I have been involved in numerous circumstances where the family was adamant that their son or daughter, husband or wife, mother or father, just wouldn't do such a horrible thing. They simply refused to believe it, even when the evidence was overwhelming and irrefutable.

As I started to review the Digman case, I couldn't help but wonder if that was the situation here. After all, navy investigators and the Riverside coroner's office had reached the same conclusion. Were the Digmans simply refusing to accept the obvious regarding their son?

Keeping that in mind, I had some immediate concerns or problems presented by the autopsy and investigative reports that caused me to see red flags right away. For starters, authorities had not tested Captain Digman's hands to determine if he had fired the handgun. This is a simple test that, if it had been conducted and shown that there was gun powder residue on his hands, would have gone a long way in convincing people that this was a suicide.

Then there was the fact that no one had ever recovered the bullet. This was astonishing. The bullet would have lodged in the ceiling or wall of the house somewhere, yet authorities didn't take the initiative to find it. Why does it matter that they didn't find the bullet? If they had recovered the bullet, they could have tested it to prove that it was the bullet that killed Jeffrey Digman and that it had been fired from the .44 magnum.

In mid-December, I received notice that Naval Investigative Services [NIS] investigators had agreed to exhume the body of Capt. Jeffrey Digman for the purpose of conducting a second autopsy. This mere fact indicated that even the military investigators realized that their initial probe had not been thorough enough and that there were questions that needed answering. It also showed that the Digmans' persistence in pressuring the authorities to answer their questions had finally paid off.

On January 17, 1990, nearly a year after Captain Digman's death, I flew to San Diego to participate in the exhumation and second autopsy. The day before, I had received a twenty-seven-page notebook from Ted Gunderson that contained original crime scene photographs. Because I was so busy prior to my flight to San Diego, I didn't get a chance to review the photographs or the notebook until I was on the plane.

Airplane trips are a wonderful time and place for me to get work done. There are no phone calls and no secretaries to interrupt me. And it's not like I can do much else other than sleep, watch the silly in-flight videos, or do my work. That being said, I am always careful about not displaying work materials too much. The photographs are, many times, extremely graphic or gory. They are of crime scenes or autopsies, which most people simply do not want to see. So I try to hold them in a position where the person seated next to me on the plane does not have to witness them.

The photographs depicted Digman lying on his queen-sized bed in his bedroom. Nightstands with lamps were on both sides of the bed. The bed had two pillows, white sheets, and a blanket covering it. The sheets and blanket on the bed were pulled down at an angle as if one person had slept in the bed the night before. The other side of the bed was unruffled.

The walls were bare of posters or pictures. There were blood or tissue stains on the walls and on the nightstand on the far side of the bed. There was a large bullet hole in the ceiling near the far side of the wall. I verified in the reports that the bullet had never been recovered, which as I have indicated was unusual.

Jeffrey was wearing a blue shirt and black jeans. He was lying in a supine position on his bed facing the ceiling. His arms were by his sides. His head rested on the white sheets, which were soaked in his blood.

In the photographs, I noticed an abrasion clearly visible near his right upper cheekbone. I wondered why the Riverside coroner had not mentioned this in his report. Was this an injury or bruise that was caused at the time of his death or much earlier? I just didn't know, but I made a note to ask about it.

Jeffrey's body was lying across the top half of the bed with his legs and feet dangling to the floor. The .44-caliber magnum was lying between his legs on the floor, with the muzzle resting in a blood-drenched portion of the carpet.

In two of the photographs, I noticed that Captain Digman's right thumb was sticking up, and it was blue. That didn't make sense to me. The only reason his thumb would have been blue would have been due to the postmortem settling of the blood, also known as lividity. However, the blood would have settled in the thumb only if Digman's thumb had been pointing down, not up. This just didn't fit.

I also spent about an hour of the five-hour flight reviewing the original autopsy and investigative reports. The autopsy reports from the Riverside officials and the military seemed to be written so as to contend that this was a suicide, ignoring any points that seemed contradictory. Maybe this was because all the evidence indeed pointed to suicide. Or maybe the autopsy could have been less sloppily prepared.

The toxicology report was disturbing. Digman's blood-alcohol level was .24—nearly triple the legal driving limit in California. The report noted that there were five empty bottles of beer found next to his bed. Alcohol mixed with depression can be a deadly combination. Excessive alcohol has been known to encourage emotionally distraught people to act in irresponsible ways. However, a .24 blood-alcohol level for a young healthy Marine who was a frequent drinker probably wasn't that significant in and of itself.

Finally, I spent some time reviewing the comments made to family and police by Digman's friends, neighbors, and colleagues. As I noted earlier, the picture painted of Jeffrey was not entirely rosy. He had had problems. Several people thought he drank too much. His roommate and a former girlfriend said that Jeffrey would work all day, exercise, then retreat to his bedroom, where he drank alone and watched television all evening. He didn't enjoy going to parties or meeting new people.

He was also obsessive about his new home. He kept the house meticulously clean and was frequently upset at Major Wood for not doing the same.

But the primary focus of the comments from friends, neighbors, and colleagues regarded Jeffrey's being reassigned to Puerto Rico. It was clear that he was unhappy about it. A next-door neighbor said Jeffrey had talked to her about suicide and how he hated that he was being forced to spend two years in Puerto Rico. "He seemed very troubled to me," the neighbor told police.

The best insight into Jeffrey's life and thought processes was the thirty-page summary written by Jeffrey's mother, Donna. In it she admits that her son was not happy about being reassigned to Puerto Rico. However, she said that in the days just before he shipped out, "he did not show any signs of severe depression or exhibit any bizarre behavior."

"Jeffrey told me the day before he left that he was not really happy about going to Puerto Rico," Donna wrote. "I asked him if he would be okay, and he assured me he would. He was upset, but he was clearly not suicidal."

Interestingly, the Digmans said that once their son moved to Puerto Rico, he made some new friends. He had told them it wasn't as bad as he had thought it would be, even though he continued to worry about the condition of his house. In fact, Jeffrey told them about meeting Lucy Garcia. He told his parents that he and Lucy had spent the Christmas holiday together and were even thinking about renting an apartment together.

In statements to authorities and later to news reporters, Lucy said that she talked with Jeffrey just a few days before he died and that he "seemed totally normal."[7] "He was his usual self, talking about the things we were going to do when he got back," she said.[8]

But Lucy also admitted that Jeffrey had a dark, disturbing side. "Jeffrey was acting strange at times," she told Donna Digman in a telephone conversation. "He seemed preoccupied with something that he was not talking to me about. Jeffrey would play "Moon River" over and over, sometimes as often as fifty times a night."[9]

The last person anyone knows of who spoke to Jeffrey before his death was Gema Pfieffer, a friend of his in San Diego. She chatted with him about fifty minutes before he died. She said that she offered to take him to the airport that evening to catch the red-eye flight back to Puerto Rico. He declined, saying that he already had a ride.

"Jeffrey sounded completely normal," said Pfieffer. "Definitely not suicidal."[10]

Ted Gunderson picked me up at my hotel early the next morning to take me to the Balboa Naval Hospital where the autopsy was to be performed. There were eleven people present at the second autopsy, including four military investigators, the Riverside coroner, Ted Gunderson, Dr. Brian Peterson, myself, and three others.

The body had been exhumed the day before and was brought in to us still in the standard military casket. The body was fully clothed with the dress blue uniform. Resting on his chest was a decomposed flower in a plastic wrapper. Captain Digman held a gold-colored metal cross on a chain in his white gloved hands.

Despite being underground for nearly a year, the body was in good shape with very little decay. The clothes were removed. There was a heavy brownish green mold that had developed on his hands. I noticed an Eagle tattoo on his right upper arm.

We started the examination by focusing on the entrance wound at the right temporal area—about 3.5 centimeters above the top of the right ear. Dr. Peterson, who was conducting the autopsy, shaved the hair around the wound. I was surprised that the Riverside pathologists who conducted the initial autopsy a year earlier had not done so. In a case such as this, shaving the hair away allows us to examine the wound more closely. We saw that the wound was fairly circular in shape and well circumscribed. There was no stippling pattern.

This was the first of the facts that did not fit with suicide. The entrance wound was not the typical star-shaped wound on the side of the head that we see in most suicide cases. If you shoot yourself and the muzzle is held firmly against your head, the gases have no room to explode once outside of the muzzle of the gun. Instead, they are pushed into the skin through the bullet hole and then they explode beneath the skin. That causes a star-shaped configuration or a jagged laceration on the skin. That was not the situation here. It was a more circular hole, which meant the muzzle was close but had not been held directly against the skin.

Most people who commit suicide press the muzzle of the gun against the skin. That would especially be true for someone who wasn't using his naturally strong, favored hand. He would rest it or press it against the skin to steady or support the gun. That's not to say that Captain Digman could not have shot himself by holding the gun away from his head; he could have. But the great majority of suicides caused by a gunshot wound to the head have the star-shaped, or irregular, jagged laceration.

Just as Digman's allegedly using his right hand did not disprove suicide, neither did the absence of the stippling pattern. But it did raise another doubt in my mind.

The autopsy continued.

Digman's nose was intact and straight, with no apparent injuries. However, we did take note of a reddish abrasion and contusion or cut on the lateral right cheek—the one I had noticed in the photographs earlier. His teeth were intact, held together with white string.

On the left side of the victim's head was the exit wound. There was no stippling, no soot deposit, and no surrounding abrasion. The wound was straight up from the back border of the left ear. It was slightly higher on the head than the entrance wound. And it was larger than the entrance wound, which is typical of exit wounds.

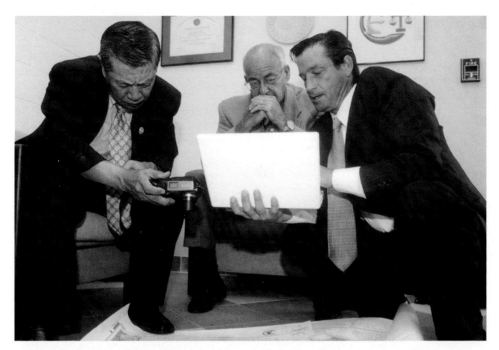

Attorney Matt Dalton briefs forensics experts Dr. Henry Lee and Dr. Cyril Wecht on the Scott Peterson case at the forensics lab in Ripon, California. Credit: Polaris Images/Debbie Noda

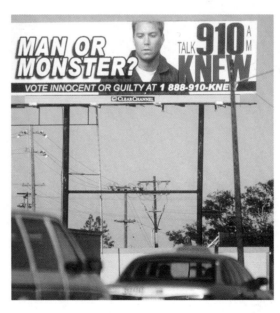

A radio station billboard in Redwood, California, asks callers to vote on the guilt or innocence of Scott Peterson in the deaths of his wife and unborn son. Credit: AP Photo/Paul Sakuma

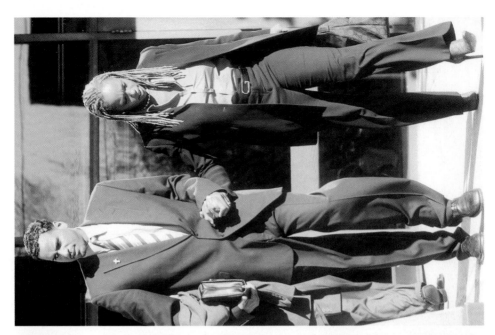

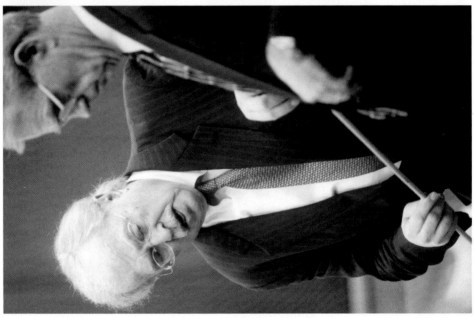

Left: Dr. Michael Baden shows the shotgun blast trajectory during his testimony with Jayson Williams's defense attorney, Joseph Hayden, on March 24, 2004.
Credit: AP Photo/Ed Pagliarini

Right: Jayson Williams and his wife, Tanya, leave the Somerset County Courthouse in Somerville, New Jersey, after the second day of jury deliberations on April 28, 2004.
Credit: AP

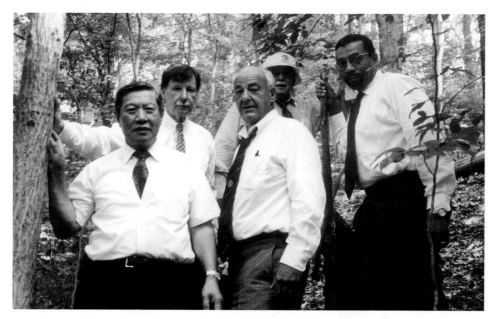

The Levy family attorney, Billy Martin *(far right)*, brings his team of experts to the site where Chandra Levy's body was found: *(from left)* forensics expert Dr. Henry Lee; investigator Joseph McCann; Dr. Cyril Wecht; forensics expert Dr. Michael Baden. Credit: Courtesy of Dr. Henry Lee

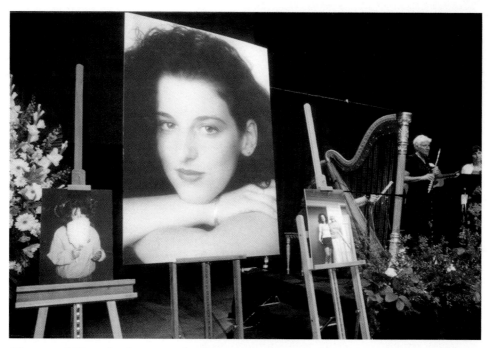

Photos of Chandra Levy on display at her memorial service on Tuesday, May 28, 2002, at Modesto Centre Plaza. Credit: AP Photo/Debbie Noda

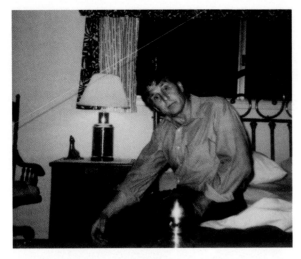

Bill Digman seated where his son, Jeffrey, was allegedly seated when he shot himself in the head. The string above Bill's head was the actual path of the bullet that killed Jeffrey. Credit: From the files of Dr. Cyril Wecht

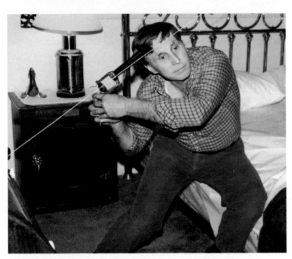

As part of a reenactment, Bill Digman aligned the pistol with the actual trajectory of the bullet. This showed that Jeffrey would have to have been standing in a highly unlikely position to have shot himself. Credit: From the files of Dr. Cyril Wecht

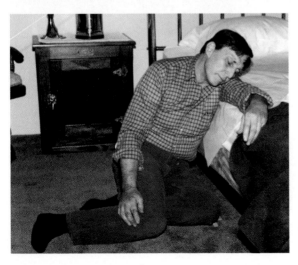

The reconstruction of the shooting demonstrated that Jeffrey's body would have collapsed on the floor, next to the bed—not lying on the bed faceup as he was found. Credit: From the files of Dr. Cyril Wecht

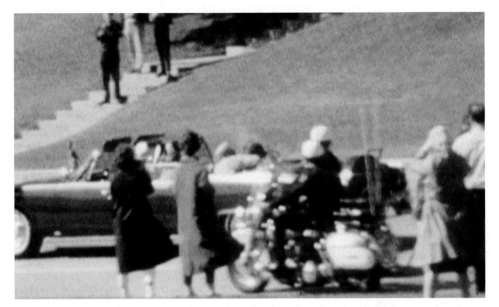

First Lady Jacqueline Kennedy cradles the head of her husband seconds after he was shot. This frame image was made from a restored version of a film showing the assassination of President John F. Kennedy. Credit: AP Photo

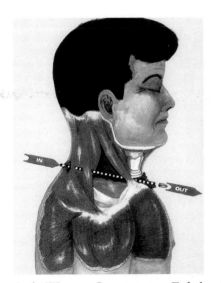
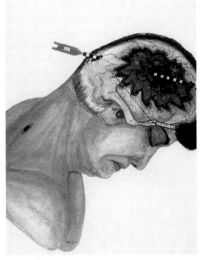

Left: Warren Commission Exhibit 385 shows a downward trajectory of the first bullet (also known as the "magic bullet") as it struck President Kennedy. However, the entrance wound depicted in this official drawing had been improperly moved up a few inches from the back into the neck in order to meet the path the bullet would have had to take for it to exit at the bullet wound in the front of the neck. *Right:* The Warren Commission, in Exhibit 388, concluded the fatal bullet struck President Kennedy at the base of the rear of his skull and exited the right side of his head.

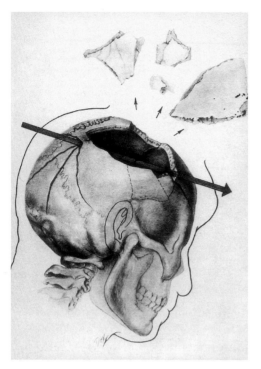

The House Select Committee on Assassinations, in volume 7, page 125, concluded the fatal bullet struck JFK four inches higher on the skull than the Warren Commission concluded. The exact location of the entrance wounds on JFK's head remains a controversial matter forty-two years later.

Dr. McClelland's Drawing

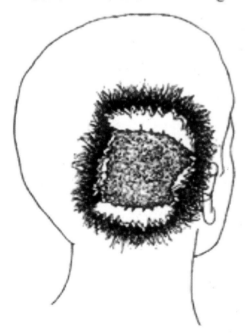

Assassinations Records and Review Board #264 is a drawing by Dr. McClelland, an emergency room physician who treated JFK at Parkland Hospital, showing where he saw JFK's head wound, which was much lower on the back right of the head.

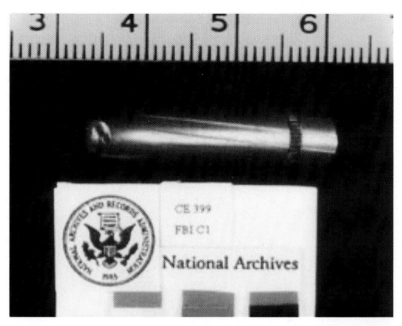

Warren Commission Exhibit CE 399, also known as the "magic bullet."

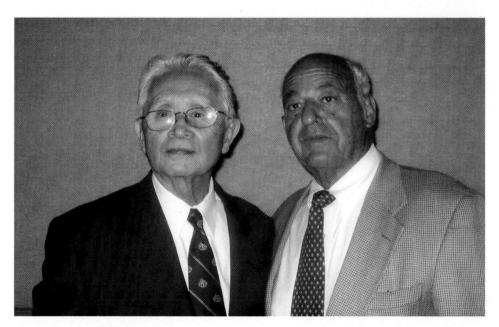

Dr. Tom Noguchi and I met not long after he performed the autopsy on
Marilyn Monroe. We have been close friends and colleagues ever since. As
Chief Medical Examiner of Los Angeles, he consulted me in such cases as
Robert Kennedy, the Charles Manson murders of Sharon Tate and the La
Biancas, and the kidnapping of Patty Hearst by the Symbionese Liberation
Army. Credit: From the files of Dr. Noguchi and Dr. Wecht

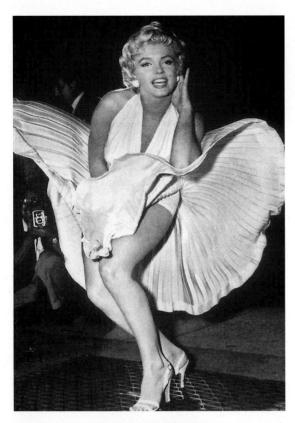

Marilyn Monroe in character for *The Seven Year Itch*, in one of her most famous photos, as she poses over a New York City subway grate. Credit: AP Photo/Matty Zimmerman

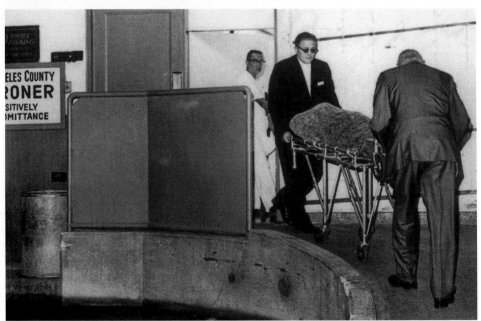

The body of Marilyn Monroe is wheeled from the Los Angeles County Morgue on August 16, 1962. Credit: AP Photo

The bullet had traveled right to left, at a slight upward angle, from front to back.

We also discovered three other injuries or wounds that had not been mentioned in the initial autopsy. There was a reddish brown lesion on Captain Digman's forehead, a contusion (a bruise) on his right elbow, and a contusion on his left middle finger. These injuries or wounds most certainly could have been the result of a struggle or altercation the night of his death, especially in the absence of any other explanation. At the very minimum, they were injuries that were completely unexplained by authorities.

Otherwise there was very little disparity in the two autopsies. This was not one of the occasions where the second autopsy disproved suicide. There was no overwhelming evidence produced during the autopsy that the gun had actually been fired from a significant distance.

That being said, troubling new questions arose from the autopsy. One of the most important questions was the angle or track of the bullet. We now had precise information regarding the angle that the bullet had taken from the time it left the chamber of the handgun, entered the temporal area of the head, traveled through the brain, and exited the opposite side of the head just above the ear.

The autopsy took less than two hours. It was clear to me that the Riverside coroner was not going to change his mind about this being a suicide. Even so, we thanked everyone for allowing us to participate and agreed to share our final reports with each other.

Now I wanted to visit the crime scene. I wanted to see the room where Jeffrey Digman allegedly took his own life. I don't visit every crime scene. In fact, I seldom do. But sometimes it helps to understand what happened if I can reenact the final few minutes or replay it in my mind.

Ted Gunderson and I met the Digmans for the first time later that day. They agreed to walk us through their son's home. Bill Digman was a retired engineer, a man in his early sixties who had remained in good physical condition. Donna was a real estate agent. It was clear from the moment that I met them that they had loved their son so much that they would do whatever was required to find out the truth.

"We just want to know what happened," Bill explained to me. "If the evidence shows us that he committed suicide, then so be it. We can't change that. We will have to live with that. But if the evidence shows otherwise, that someone else was involved or that our son was murdered, then we can't simply stand around and do nothing. We owe him that much."[11]

"I didn't drag that boy of mine to the orthodontist and to Little League practices and games to have him buried at age thirty," Donna told me, half in tears and half in anger. "They are not just going to throw him away. To the rest of the world, Jeffrey may have been this strong, courageous Marine. But to me, he will always be my little boy."

Bill told me that his son was either a victim of murder or the victim of an uncaring, neglecting Marine Corp. "I just want to know the truth," he told me. "It doesn't matter much how much it costs me or what I have to do, we must find out what happened to our son."

Donna told me about one of the last conversations she had with her son during his two-week visit back home. "I asked him how he was feeling about Puerto Rico," she said. "He told me it was all right, but he had been to places he liked better."

"In fact, I've been thinking about getting out of the military," Jeffrey had said, according to his mother.

"Don't you like what you're doing?" she asked.

"Yeah, but . . ."

Donna said that there was a long pause.

"Is it too hard?" she asked.

"No, probably too easy," he answered.

"What makes you want to get out?" Donna asked him.

"Well, I really don't," he said, after another lengthy pause.

Then came a statement from Jeffrey that Donna said had stuck with her since: "No one is going to take my captain's bars away from me."

Donna said she didn't push him further and Jeffrey volunteered no additional information. Neither Donna nor Bill seemed to know what that meant.

The couple led us to their son's second-floor bedroom. It was preserved in a way to replicate the night of the death. The blood-stained sheets were gone, of course, taken by authorities as part of their investigation. But the Digmans had replaced them with new sheets that outlined their son's body as he lay on the bed. Right before my eyes, Bill Digman and Ted Gunderson reenacted the shooting as it would have happened under the coroner's theory of suicide.

Bill sat sideways on the edge of the bed, as the Riverside coroner and military police contended that his son had done the night he shot himself. He held in his hand a .44-caliber magnum handgun, identical to the one found between his son's legs. Taking into account the entrance and exit wounds we had examined earlier that day, we projected the trajectory of the bullet using white string. (*See the photos in the insert.*)

A problem emerged. The bullet entered the ceiling at a very steep thirty-five-degree angle. If Digman had been sitting on the bed, the bullet would have entered the wall, not the ceiling, which was ten feet two inches above the floor.

Because the bullet had entered the ceiling, we decided to work backward to see where Digman must have been standing or sitting when the bullet entered his head, exited his head, and traveled into the ceiling. What we discovered was that, in order for the bullet to match the anatomically demonstrated trajectory, Jeffrey would have had to be sitting with only his left buttock on the very edge of the bed, leaning away from the bed, with his head leaning at a steep right angle. If Jeffrey shot himself in this contorted position, then, yes, the trajectories would match. But why would someone who is about to kill himself do so in such a contorted position?

Moreover, that raised another problem: Jeffrey's body, from his hips upward, was found lying faceup on the bed. If he had been in the contorted position when he was shot, his body would have fallen either completely onto the floor or only partially onto the bed. If Digman had shot himself, he would have collapsed immediately. He could not have continued to stand up on his own.

Once again, the physical facts just didn't fit.

On my flight back home to Pittsburgh that evening, I reviewed the autopsy findings, investigative reports, and crime scene photographs one more time, in an effort to piece it all together, to see if I had missed something. Looking over the photographs of Jeffrey's body on the bed, I noticed two things that the Digmans had mentioned to me.

First, there was a stream of blood flowing in a straight line down Digman's ear, down his shoulder, down his arm, and down the left side of his neck and onto his chest. It is not unusual that blood would flow from the ear following a gunshot wound to the head. Blood emanating from the ear indicates that there was an intracranial fracture (a fracture at the base of the skull) and hemorrhaging. What was unusual was the direction of the blood flow. The blood flow indicated that Digman's body was in an upright position for several seconds while the blood flowed down his body. This meant that he probably fell next to the bed in a sitting position or that at least something was holding his body upright, allowing the blood to flow in that position. If Digman had fallen straight back onto the bed after he shot himself, the blood would have run from the front to the back of his head, not from top to bottom.

There would be only one explanation for this: Digman's body was moved and placed on the bed in the position that it was found. That would also explain the trajectory or path of the bullet.

Interestingly, photographed next to Digman's bed was a paper bag with a six-pack of Budweiser beer in it. Bill and Donna told me that their son liked warm beer and that he seldom put his beer in the refrigerator. But what was strange was that one of the bottles of beer was missing. Even the first police officer at the crime scene had made a note of the missing beer bottle. The police had searched the trash cans in the house and garage but did not find the missing bottle of beer.

Bill Digman told me that he believed the missing bottle was taken by the person who killed his son. He also told me that they had found the writing desk in their son's bedroom had its hinges torn off and that a small safe that their son had kept inside was missing.

On January 26, 1990, the forensic pathologists for the navy filed their autopsy protocol on the second autopsy. Their report read: "The cause of death of Jeffrey Digman is a loose contact type gunshot wound of the head. The findings of the second autopsy examination are consistent with the initial findings that the manner of death is suicide."

The final word on this case rested with the federal medical examiner. Most people do not even realize that there is a federal medical examiner. They know their local city or county has a coroner or medical examiner. And most people are aware that the Armed Forces Institute of Pathology has numerous forensic pathologists working for it. But the federal government, after the fiasco caused by the assassination of President John F. Kennedy, created the position of federal medical examiner to review the deaths of people in which the military or federal law enforcement had jurisdiction.

The death of Jeffrey Digman fell under two jurisdictions—the Riverside coroner's office, which was never going to reopen its probe, and the federal medical examiner because it was a military death on US soil.

The federal medical examiner in 1990 was Dr. Richard Froede, whom I knew from my days in the air force in the early 1960s when he had been at the Armed Forces Institute of Pathology. He had since retired from the air force and moved to Arizona, where he spent several years as the state medical examiner. Then he was appointed as the first federal medical examiner.

Not only was Dr. Froede an excellent forensic pathologist, he was also very open and approachable. I had written to Dr. Froede about the case, requesting permission to discuss my findings and opinions with him. To his great credit, Dr. Froede agreed. In April 1989 he and I had a lengthy telephone conversation in which we reviewed all the different points of controversy or contention in the investigation. He ended the phone call by agreeing to review the entire matter.

I also sent to Dr. Froede a four-page report written on July 26, 1990, by respected criminalist Stephan A. Schliebe, who was the director of the California Laboratory of Forensic Science in Tustin. Stephan had also reconstructed the events surrounding Jeffrey Digman's death. His work on the case in the area of bullet trajectory was far more detailed than my own. He found that if Digman had been sitting on his bed when he shot himself, as Riverside authorities contended, the path of the bullet would have been ten inches above his head.

He also noted the photographs showing blood streaming down Digman's ears, saying they indicated that he was upright for several seconds after receiving the head wound. "The shot through the victim's head would most certainly have caused him to collapse instantaneously," Stephan stated in his report. "How, then, could the victim have been upright for the amount of time needed to explain the blood flow? A reasonable possibility is that someone prevented him from falling after being shot. A second possible explanation is that after the victim had been positioned on the bed, he was raised or lifted to a sitting position for a short period of time and then laid back down."

I completely agree with his assessment.

But Mr. Schliebe made an additional finding that had totally escaped me. He found evidence of blood smears on the edge of the sheet above and to the left of the victim's head. "It's an obvious contact-type transfer of blood," Stephan said. "It is not a splatter bloodstain. If the victim fell on the bed in the position he was found, how did this stain get there? The only reasonable explanation at this time is that some other individual made contact with the edge of the sheet."[12]

Again, more evidence pointing to someone else being in the room and more evidence that did not add up to this being suicide.

At the end of his investigation, Schliebe concluded that "there is a variety of physical evidence associated with this crime scene that counterindicates Jeffrey Digman died by suicide. This assemblage of evidence can reasonably be evaluated in such a way as to indicate that Jeffrey Digman struggled with someone, was either accidentally or purposely shot, and was then placed on the bed."[13]

On February 22, 1991, Dr. Froede wrote Bill Digman a two-page letter stating that he was officially reclassifying the manner of death in their son's case to "undetermined."

The Digmans never convinced the military or Riverside authorities to reopen the investigation. The truth about what happened in Jeffrey Digman's bedroom the night of January 22, 1989, might never be known. But Dr. Froede's reclassification was a huge moral victory for the family. The thought that the military for whom their son served so valiantly had listed his death as suicidal was intolerable. So they didn't stand for it. They spent several years of their lives and more than $100,000 in legal costs fighting for the truth.

What really happened to Captain Digman? Was he murdered? Did he commit suicide?

The Riverside authorities and navy investigators pointed to Jeffrey's depressed state as one of the primary reasons they believe that he killed himself. It is unquestionably true that he was upset about being reassigned to Puerto Rico. And he was unhappy about being away from his house. However, it appeared from others that he was starting to adapt. He had developed a few close friendships and had even found a girlfriend.

The statements by friends that Jeffrey was a loner, that he drank too much, that he was depressed, and that he had just watched the suicide scene in *Full Metal Jacket* are disturbing. These statements make it clear that Jeffrey probably did suffer from depression. Those things by themselves may not prove that Jeffrey was suicidal, but it is understandable how the military viewed them more strongly in light of the possibility that he was found with a seemingly self-inflicted gunshot wound. Trying to recapture the captain's state of mind was not only acceptable for the investigators, it was necessary.

But where the military and coroner's investigation totally failed was in examining the physical, medical, and forensic evidence itself. The investigation was horribly weak. They forgot to test the hands of the deceased for powder residue. They didn't find and test the bullet in the ceiling of Digman's house to see if it was the one that killed him. The investigators seemed to ignore any evidence that pointed away from suicide.

To this day, there are significant unanswered questions about this case—questions that raise doubt about its being a suicide. For example:

(1) There's the blue thumb, indicating that the body had been moved.
(2) There's the blood flow down his ear, indicating the victim was sitting or standing up for several seconds following the shooting.
(3) There's the lack of a star-shaped or jagged pattern near the entrance wound, indicating that the muzzle of the gun was not resting on the temple as it was fired.
(4) There's the fact that the gunshot was on the right side of the head when the deceased was left-handed.
(5) There's the previously undocumented injuries to Captain Digman's cheek, elbow, and finger.

But the most important evidence of all is that involving the trajectory of the bullet. It simply didn't match up with the suicide theory. There is no way scientifically for the bullet to have entered and exited Jeffrey Digman's head at the trajectory that we know it did, and for it to end up in the ceiling where we know it did, and for Digman to have landed on the bed, faceup, as he apparently did.

Forensically, medically, scientifically impossible.

Does that mean that Jeffrey was murdered?

There are three options in this case.

Number one, he was murdered and his body arranged to make it look like a suicide.

Number two, he was killed accidentally or in self-defense, and the other person involved arranged Digman's body to make it look as though he killed himself.

Number three, Digman did commit suicide, but the person who found his body panicked and placed Digman on the bed.

Of course, there could be an explanation none of us has pondered. But the fact is that the hard evidence points away from a suicide more than it does toward a suicide. Unfortunately for Jeffrey's family, unless there is some deathbed confession from the real killer, this case will probably forever be listed as "undetermined."

"Jeffrey always wanted to be a soldier," Donna Digman told me the last time I talked with her. "He loved being a Marine officer. He would have died for his country if he had been asked. It's just a shame that his country didn't stand up for him in his death."[14]

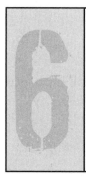

GANDER AIR CRASH

ICE OR SABOTAGE?

On December 11, 1985, a group of 248 American soldiers boarded an Egyptian Air 737 in the Sinai headed for home. Most were members of the US Army's elite Third Battalion, 502nd Infantry of the 101st Airborne, who had spent the previous five months in the Middle East. They had not been there to fight a war but to keep the peace. The soldiers were part of the Multinational Force and Observers that had the mission of implementing security protocols outlined in the peace treaty that had been signed by Israel and Egypt in 1979.

Now, as the holidays approached, they were gleeful to be headed home. As they marched toward the plane that would begin their journey back to America, the soldiers in unison sang a well-known military tune: "We have a rendezvous with destiny . . ."[1]

Little did they know how true that statement was.

Their flight home, to their base at Fort Campbell, Kentucky, was a two-day journey. The first stop was Cairo International Airport in Egypt, where they would switch planes. While the government of Egypt was considered an ally of the United States, the city of Cairo was a known serious security risk for Americans. It was also a stronghold for the Islamic fundamentalist group the Muslim Brotherhood. Because the layover would last for several hours, the soldiers were allowed to explore the city. However, they were required to wear civilian clothes so as not to invoke attacks.[2]

Several hours later, the soldiers boarded the jetliner that would carry them home—Arrow Air Flight 950, a DC-8 chartered by the US Army to transport its soldiers to and from the Middle East. A sole Egyptian soldier assigned to guard the plane watched as other Egyptian soldiers loaded the cargo, including six coffin-sized boxes. The crates were so heavy that they caused the plane to be overweight. As a result, forty-one soldiers were required to leave their duffle bags behind. This was highly unusual because soldiers are seldom, if ever, separated from their gear.[3]

At 10:30 PM, eight hours behind scheduled, Flight 950 departed Cairo for Cologne, Germany, where the plane would undergo one last refueling before making the transatlantic trip.

The Arrow Air jet landed at the Gander International Airport in Newfoundland, Canada, just before dawn at 5:34 AM. This was to be the final refueling stop before arriving at Fort Campbell. Many of the soldiers, excited about being hours away from home, called family and friends from the airport's pay phones, letting them know they were safe in our neighboring country and would soon be home for the holidays. The soldiers had an hour to enjoy a cup of coffee, shop in the duty-free store for Christmas gifts, and buy candy bars.[4]

Several of the soldiers bought T-shirts that read: "I Survived Gander."

The plane was cleared for takeoff by air traffic control at 6:44 AM: "Big A 950. Gander Tower. Cleared for takeoff on twenty-two. Winds are calm."[5]

Air traffic control officials in the tower reported the plane's roll out and departure appeared completely normal and without any reports of problems. The jetliner taxied down the ten thousand-foot runway and into the sky, which was just beginning to show its first signs of morning.

Less than two minutes later, an approaching plane sent a radio transmission to air traffic control: "Tower, its Flight 351. You seem to have an explosion off here to the west here."[6]

About one-half mile after lifting off from runway twenty-two, Arrow Air Flight 950 crashed into a wooden area between the Trans-Canada Highway and Gander Lake. Firefighters and rescue workers immediately responded to emergency calls. But they were hampered by the rugged terrain and the intense heat generated from the burning jet fuel.

Parts of the plane's fuselage, the cargo, and human remains were scattered for hundreds of yards. Firefighters battled the blaze for four hours before finally getting it under control. It took nearly thirty hours before the fire was completely extinguished.[7]

I remember learning about the horrific air crash as I prepared to head to work at the Allegheny County coroner's office the morning of December 12. The tragedy was the lead news story for CNN and the early morning news shows, such as *The Today Show* and *Good Morning America*. The news stated that 256 people—248 soldiers and eight members of the plane's crew—had been onboard the plane that crashed and that there were no survivors. The television news reporters called it the worst US military crash in history, in terms of loss of life.

By 10:30 AM, as firefighters continued to battle the blaze, US officials announced that ice on the wings of the jet was suspected to be the cause for the crash. A Pentagon spokesperson immediately downplayed any thoughts or suggestions that a bomb or terrorist attack played any role in the catastrophe.

The investigation of the crash was hampered by a severe snowstorm that hit the area a few days after the crash. The snowstorm was so bad, in fact, that the entire search of the crash site was put on hold for weeks.

I learned later that day that fourteen of the young men aboard the plane were from the Pittsburgh area. It was truly a national tragedy, exacerbated by the fact that it happened during the holiday season. These were young men and women who were dedicated to serving their country and making the world a safer place. They had put their lives at risk for the rest of us and had been on their way home to see their loved ones.

At a heart-wrenching memorial service a few days later at Fort Campbell, President Ronald Reagan met with the families of each of the deceased soldiers. No matter your political affiliation, most Americans found the former president to be a likable fellow whose speeches could comfort even the most distraught. I recall seeing his speech live on CNN that day. And I especially remember a few key words he spoke to the families: "We wonder, how could this be?" he asked. "How could it have happened and why?"

At the time, I didn't give a second thought as to the cause of the crash. Leading authorities of both Canada and the United States were strongly asserting that an icing of the wings was the key factor.

The explanation seemed totally plausible to me. After all, it was December in Newfoundland. It had to be cold. And I remembered the news stories that the severe snowstorm had hit Gander right after the crash. So ice on the wings seemed a likely cause of the crash.

Nearly three years passed and I didn't really give much more thought to the tragedy, except for reading the occasional article in the newspaper on the anniversary of the crash or hearing some group or organization's claim that the cause of the crash was something other than ice.

On October 28, 1988, the Canadian Aviation Safety Board, the nine-member governmental agency charged with investigating and determining the official cause of the crash, issued its 112-page report. The report, concluding that wing icing was responsible for the disaster, stated:

> The Canadian Aviation Safety Board was unable to determine the exact sequence of events which led to this accident. The

Board believes, however, that the weight of the evidence supports the conclusion that, shortly after lift-off, the aircraft experienced an increase in drag and reduction in the lift which
resulted in a stall at low altitude from which recovery was not
possible. The most probable cause of the stall was determined to
be ice contamination on the leading edge and upper surface of
the wing. Other possible factors such as loss of thrust from the
number four engine and inappropriate take-off reference speeds
may have compounded the effects of the contamination.[8]

I, probably like most Americans, believed that was the end of
it. Investigation over, case closed. After all, why would the US
government want or need to mislead the American public about
the cause of an airplane crash? Furthermore, what would motivate
Canadian officials to participate in such a cover-up?

The Gander crash didn't cross my mind again until eighteen
months later, in early March 1990. That's when prominent Pittsburgh television journalist Terri Taylor, of KDKA Channel 2, contacted me. Terri, who had interviewed me previously for an assort-
ment of stories she had done on an array of deaths in the Pittsburgh
area, had been conducting an investigation into the Gander crash.

Earlier that year, several families of the soldiers who had died
contacted Terri saying things just weren't adding up. She told me
that many of the families were told by military officials that they
would not be allowed to see their loved ones' autopsy reports. I
agreed that this seemed rather outrageous.

Terri had also traveled to Newfoundland where she interviewed key witnesses to the crash, as well as Canadian investigators involved in the official inquiry.

"The evidence just doesn't seem to support the official line
about ice on the wings causing this crash," Terri told me on the
telephone. "And the way the federal government, especially the
FBI and the army, have been acting, it certainly seems like they're
hiding something. They certainly are not being very forthcoming."

Terri told me that she had interviewed Vice President Dan

Quayle about the subject, but he claimed that he didn't know much. "There's a shock," I told her sarcastically. She laughed and agreed.

However, Terri told me that lawyers for her television station had filed an official public records request with the federal government under the Freedom of Information Act, seeking copies of any medical or autopsy reports regarding the soldiers who died. The legal fight to obtain the death records already had been long and heated between the families and the military.

To bolster their case to have the records released, Terri asked if I would be willing to prepare and file an official affidavit to be submitted to the FBI and the Armed Forces Institute of Pathology (AFIP), stating why it was important that the records be made public and what information could be gleaned from the documents. The AFIP was the official federal government agency for identifying bodies and conducting autopsies or other medicolegal examinations or tests.

Let me state this up front: I have tremendous respect for the AFIP. The AFIP, which was created following World War II, is the mecca of forensic pathology. My relationship with the AFIP dates back to 1960 and 1961, when I served as a pathologist at Maxwell Air Force Base in Alabama. I would attend seminars on forensic pathology at the AFIP. Later in my career, I lectured at the AFIP and have become an official consultant to the AFIP's Division of Legal Medicine. I have worked with the AFIP many times over the years and have great respect for many of its forensic pathologists.

"When we get the autopsy records, would you be willing to review them for us?" Terri asked.

Of course I would.

Terri told me that the television station didn't have any money to pay for my services. But I answered that what she was doing was a public service in informing the public what really happened on that day. I would be happy to file the affidavit and then review the reports once they were released and provide my opinions on a pro bono basis.

A few days later, Terri mailed me a copy of the Canadian Aviation Safety Board's (CASB) official report for the Gander crash. She also sent me a videotape of all the stories she had done on the subject. They were fascinating. A few days later, I completed the affidavit that sought access to all the autopsy and toxicology reports, as well as all microscopic slides. Two days after that, lawyers for KDKA-TV sent my affidavit to the AFIP via express, registered mail.

The CASB document Terri had mailed to me detailed the flight history of the airplane and the crew who flew it. It documented the damage to the jetliner following the crash. It examined weather conditions and the official operating procedures that pilots should follow under certain negative conditions, such as icing.

The CASB ended its report by listing thirty-two findings, including:

(1)   During the approach to land at Gander, the existing meteorological conditions were conducive to ice accretion to the leading edge of the wing.

(2)   While on the ground at Gander, the aircraft was exposed to freezing and frozen precipitation capable of producing roughening on the wing upper surface.

(3)   While the aircraft was on the ground at Gander, the difference between the wing surface temperature and the outside temperature was conducive to the formation of frost on the surface of the wing.

(4)   The aircraft was not de-iced prior to take-off.

(25)   The accident investigation into the causes and factors that led to this occurrence was severely hampered by the lack of information that a serviceable cockpit voice recorder and enhanced-capability digital flight data recorder could have provided.

(28)   The balance of the evidence did not support the occurrence of a pre-impact fire or explosion either accidental or as the result of sabotage.[9]

When I finished reviewing the official CASB report, I noticed a second document—a minority report. Before that time, I had not realized that only five of the nine members of the CASB had signed the official findings. Nor did I know that on November 14, 1988, the four remaining members of the CASB issued a dissenting report. The four, in a twenty-one-page opinion, strongly criticized the majority report.

> In our judgment, the wings of the Arrow Air DC-8 were not contaminated by ice—certainly not enough for ice contamination to be a factor in this accident. The aircraft's trajectory and performance differed markedly from that which could plausibly result from ice contamination. The aircraft did not stall. Accordingly, we cannot agree—indeed, we categorically disagree—with the major findings.
>
> The available evidence convincingly shows that the outboard engine was producing little power before it contacted the trees. The investigation of the other engines was inconclusive with regard to pre-impact status.
>
> The evidence shows that the Arrow Air DC-8 suffered an onboard fire and a massive loss of power before it crashed. But, we could not establish a direct link between the fire and the loss of power. The fire may have been associated with an in-flight detonation from an explosive or incendiary device. Consequential damage to various systems precipitated the crash.[10]

The minority report pointed out that the majority's conclusion—that ice on the wings caused the crash—was based totally on theoretical possibilities. There was no actual evidence of ice buildup on the wings. In fact, the minority report included interviews with ground crew workers at the Gander International Airport who stated that they checked the plane before takeoff and found no ice on the wings. In addition, a plane had departed from the Gander airport just an hour earlier without any report of ice on the wings.

The dissenting report also included a section that seemed to provide strong support that a fire or explosion had caused the crash. The report quoted a truck driver on the Trans-Canada Highway that morning who saw the jetliner as it was taking off. He stated that he saw a "yellow/orange glow" as if "the right-hand side of the aircraft was on fire." Seconds later, he testified, the plane crashed. The report cited a second eyewitness who saw the plane pass directly over his head. "My first impression of the glow was that it was a fire," the witness stated.[11]

The Islamic Jihad also had made four separate attempts to claim responsibility for sabotaging the plane after the crash. Remember, this is a time when terrorism against the United States was on the rise. Just two months prior to the Gander crash, in October 1985, a group of terrorists formerly with the Palestinian Liberation Organization hijacked an Italian cruise liner, the *Achille Lauro*, and threw a sixty-nine-year-old disabled New York resident overboard in his wheelchair live on national television.[12] Despite the public acknowledgment by the Islamic Jihad that they were responsible, the Reagan administration publicly rejected such a claim.

The minority report caused such a political stir in Canada that the nation's Transportation Ministry appointed retired Canadian Supreme Court justice Wilbur Estey to examine both CASB findings and to make his own report. In the end, Justice Estey, who was well respected by both sides, issued a thirty-four-page opinion on July 17, 1989, in which he concluded that there wasn't enough evidence to support the theory that ice on the wings caused the crash. But the judge also stated that he didn't think reopening the crash investigation would do any good. He reported that the evidence needed to determine conclusively what caused the crash had long been destroyed.[13]

During the next two weeks, Terri and my staff at the coroner's office provided me with various newspaper articles about the crash, the subsequent investigation, and the controversy surrounding it.

The families of dozens of the soldiers had banded together to form an organization with the goal of seeking more answers from the American and Canadian governments regarding the crash that killed their loved ones.

In a later conversation, Terri told me that she and other journalists had found some startling information in the Tower Report that led her and others to suspect that there was a connection between Iran-Contra and the Gander crash. The Tower Report was the official findings of the investigation into the Reagan administration's trading weapons in return for the release of hostages. The government panel commissioned to conduct the investigation was led by former Texas senator John Tower.

In a series of investigative news reports broadcast on KDKA and subsequently on *Investigative Reports* on the Arts & Entertainment Network (A&E), Terri's hard work and journalistic skills were evident. She and the other journalists gained reams of information from the Tower Report.

The report found that in November 1985, less than three weeks prior to the crash, Lt. Col. Oliver North made a secret deal with Iran. He agreed to covertly ship eighty Hawk missiles to Iran in return for Iranian leaders obtaining the release of five Americans being held hostage by Islamic terrorist groups. One of the hostages being negotiated was Associated Press reporter Terry Anderson.[14]

The secret deal was a major breach of official US policy, which stated that the nation would never negotiate with terrorists. The secret trade was scheduled to take place on November 24, 1985, according to the Tower Report. Under the arrangement, the missiles would arrive in Tehran every two hours. As the missiles were delivered, certain hostages would be released. North's personal notes, according to the Tower Report, show that Arrow Air would play a major role either in the delivery of the missiles or in the return of the hostages.

But the transfer was never made. Iranian leaders were not happy with the types of missiles they received, according to the

Tower Report. The Iranians wanted missiles that could shoot down Iraqi aircraft. As you may recall, Iraq and Iran were at war at that time. The Hawk missiles did not have that capability. An additional slap in the face to the Iranians was that the missiles that were delivered had Israeli markings on them. Only eighteen missiles were delivered. No hostages were released.

A few days later, Iranian prime minister Mir Hussein Moussavi, who was negotiating the deal with Lieutenant Colonel North, sent an urgent message to President Reagan: "We have done everything we said we were going to do, and you are now cheating us, and you must act quickly to remedy this situation."[15]

In a memo dated December 9, 1985, Lieutenant Colonel North, apparently fearing retaliation, recommended that the missiles the Iranians wanted be sent to them. "U.S. reversal now in midstream could ignite Iranian fire, hostages would be our minimum losses," North warned in the memo. It was written three days prior to the Gander crash.[16]

Of course, the American public had no idea any of this clandestine activity was occurring. I remember watching President Reagan later on television asserting that not even he knew such an operation was underway.

Another of Terri's great scoops focused on the Federal Bureau of Investigation. According to Terri, the FBI had always stated publicly that it had never investigated the Gander crash because there was never any evidence of criminal activity or terrorism. However, KDKA obtained scores of documents through the Freedom of Information Act, including a 277-page report by the FBI. Call me crazy, but a 277-page report indicates to me that there had been some sort of FBI inquiry. However, about 95 percent of the information in the report was blacked out.

The report did show, nonetheless, that FBI agents had traveled to Miami in response to the Gander crash. Miami just happened to be the home of Arrow Air. Former Arrow Air captain Steve Saunders told Terri that an FBI agent visited him days after the Gander crash and asked him to take the agent into the belly of an Arrow Air DC-8 that was identical to the Gander plane. Saunders told KDKA that he was asked by an FBI agent about possible placement of explosives and stowaways. "He asked me if an individual would be able to survive a long flight in the lower forward baggage hole," Saunders told Terri on camera. "And I said, 'yes, he could.'"[17]

Terri also scored an interview with a key member of the ground crew who had been on duty at Gander International Airport the morning of December 12, 1985. He emphatically disputed that there was any ice on the wings.

In early June, I was contacted by the AFIP and told that I would be given access to the information that I had requested. However, the AFIP limited access only to me as a forensic pathologist. Unfortunately, Terri was prohibited from joining me.

I arrived midmorning at the Armed Forces Institute of Pathology headquarters, which is based at Walter Reed Hospital in Silver Springs, Maryland, a suburb of Washington, DC. Prior to examining the Gander autopsy records, I visited with several friends and colleagues.

Then, I settled in for several hours of reading and study.

My first task was to review the protocol that had been used in recovering and examining the remains. AFIP officials had arrived in Gander about eight hours after the crash. Their mission was to help recover and prepare the bodies for examination. By the end of the first day, approximately 125 bodies had been recovered and moved to a special hangar at Gander International Airport, which was turned into a temporary morgue. By December 15 the recovery team announced it had located all the remains.

For some reason, Canadian officials agreed on December 14 to allow the bodies to be flown to Dover Air Force Base, where the AFIP would conduct all the pathological and toxicological examinations. To this day, I do not understand why the CASB did not want or demand that the bodies be autopsied there in Gander under its control and supervision. Canada had jurisdiction; the

United States did not. And it's not as if Canada is some third world country lacking expertise in forensic pathology. It is understandable that the Reagan administration or the military would have wanted the bodies of the soldiers returned to the United States as quickly as possible. But the US officials should have allowed the Canadian investigators to do their jobs.

The transfer of the bodies began on December 16 and was completed within two days. The task of the AFIP was twofold: identify the remains and examine each body and body part.

Each body was weighed and placed on a gurney. A volunteer carrying a packet of medical information was assigned to each body and stayed with the body throughout the process. This assured officials that the correct postmortem medical and dental records stayed with the appropriate remains and that the remains were not misplaced or neglected. Each body was photographed before being transferred to the next area.

The FBI team then fingerprinted the remains. Each body was x-rayed for medical and dental purposes. Copies were provided to the FBI agents who assisted with the identification process.

Finally, the bodies were sent to the autopsy area, where forensic pathologists conducted complete examinations and performed toxicology tests. By December 22 all autopsies had been completed. The army estimated that it had used medical and dental records as well as fingerprinting to identify 80 percent of the soldiers. Once the remains were identified, the bodies were embalmed and placed in caskets for shipping.

To me, this process seemed not only reasonable, but the model of efficiency. It was obvious to me that the AFIP was well prepared for such a crisis. And they appeared to handle it extremely well. I read an article later in the *Army Times* in which a medical doctor in the army's Central Identification Laboratory claimed that as many as 35 percent of the Gander crash victims had been misidentified. However, I never heard any more about those allegations and have no idea if they were true.

I turned my focus to the autopsy examinations, which were extremely brief but to the point. Each record listed the soldier's name, rank, hometown, and weight. Each autopsy also listed, as the cause of death, the plane crash that caused the body to experience deadly trauma and, in some instances, dismemberment. Each report also concluded with the fact that the soldier died on impact.

However, when I studied the toxicology reports, something jumped out at me right away. The facts did not add up. I've seen a lot of weird things in my life, having performed thousands and thousands of autopsies and having investigated some of the most bizarre homicides you could ever imagine. But as I examined one toxicology report after another, I was literally stunned, befuddled, and even disturbed.

That afternoon, I boarded a plane back to Pittsburgh. I had agreed with Terri Taylor that I would not discuss my findings with anyone else before she had the opportunity to interview me.

The next morning, Terri and her television crew showed up at my office to do the on-camera interview. As her photographer was setting up the lighting and the camera, I walked Terri through my findings. She was as amazed as I was.

I started off the interview by telling Terri that there was absolutely no reason for these records to be sealed. And that was especially true if the government actually believed that ice on the wings caused the crash.

"I find it difficult to believe that they have done such a sloppy, incomplete, and negligent job unless they have been ordered to do it this way," I told KDKA. "Of course the victims' families are entitled to these reports. There's no question about it. I know it from my two years in the air force and from my decades of work with the AFIP. They are obliged by law and morality to turn these reports over to families."[18]

Then I announced the shocking revelation.

After having carefully examined the toxicology reports of the 256 soldiers and crew, I found that the carbon monoxide levels in more than four dozen of the soldiers was at 70 percent or higher—a level that is considered highly lethal.

Carbon monoxide, also known as CO, is a colorless, tasteless, odorless gas that is created by anything that burns except natural gas. Carbon monoxide can be created by car engines, cigarettes, home heating units that use fossil fuels, and burning wood, just to name a few examples. Most humans have some small levels, of about 2 or 3 percent, of CO in their systems. Cigarette smokers are known to have about 6 to 8 percent carbon monoxide in their blood. People who regularly inhale secondhand smoke have been known to have CO levels as high as 12 percent.

The problem is that carbon monoxide acts as an asphyxiant in the body. The hemoglobin molecule in our blood has a 210-times greater affinity for CO than it does for oxygen. As a result, the carbon monoxide occupies all the space in the red blood cells, which are supposed to be delivering oxygen to the brain, to the heart, and throughout the body. Without the oxygen, the body suffocates.

Carbon monoxide levels in the body can be determined by examining blood, brain tissue, or liver tissue. CO levels of 15 percent will cause the individual to develop a headache. At about 20 percent, the person experiences dizziness. If the carbon monoxide level reaches 40 or 50 percent, the body will go unconscious and probably slip into a coma. Death is nearly certain for carbon monoxide levels of 60 percent or higher.

"What does it mean that these soldiers had CO levels of 70 percent or higher? Terri asked.

"These soldiers were alive and they breathed in the carbon monoxide," I told her. "There was either a fire or something aboard the plane that emitted carbon monoxide prior to the plane crashing. These soldiers had to breathe in the CO while still onboard the plane because the autopsies show that the soldiers were dead on impact."[19]

"But with carbon monoxide levels of 70 percent or higher,

these fifty soldiers were either dead or dying before the plane crashed into the ground," I told her.

Terri then asked if it was possible for the carbon monoxide to have been inhaled by the soldiers' bodies after the crash, as they lay dead on the ground.

"There is no question whatsoever that postmortem absorption of carbon monoxide does not occur under any circumstances," I responded. "I do not care if there is a pool of blood inside an open vacuum in which carbon monoxide is being pumped, CO will not contaminate the blood."

"To get to this level, 70 or 80 percent, the person has to be alive for several seconds or maybe even a couple of minutes to breathe in this level of carbon monoxide in an environment where there is a lot of smoke," I explained. "This finding is much more consistent with there being a fire aboard Flight 950 prior to its crash."

Terri told me that the Canadians argued that there was no explosion on the plane because there was no evidence of shrapnel found in the bodies of the victims. She also said she had heard that there was a question about whether the chemical explosive Cemtex was used on Flight 950.

"You don't have to have flying shrapnel to prove or disprove an explosion," I told her. "What you look for is the presence of chemical constituents of Cemtex on the people's clothing and the seat covers and so forth. There are all kinds of tests that could be done—inspectographic, inspectophotometric, infrared, neutron activation analysis.

"Unfortunately, the evidence of Flight 950 has been destroyed," I reminded Terri. "Clothes and seat covers were burned. Pieces of the fuselage were plowed under. That is the bitter irony of this tragedy. They destroyed the evidence, thereby preventing court action or any legal proceedings. In the absence of the legal proceedings, they are not required to answer questions or conduct tests. Meanwhile the government arrogantly sits back and contends there is no proof.

"But it is the government that destroyed the proof," I continued. "This is a major scandal. I believe that while the investigation has been seriously compromised and the search for the truth has been made much more difficult, it is still possible to determine what happened simply by the government releasing the information it has."

Terri's report that included my interview aired on KDKA on Friday, June 8, 1990. On March 20, 1992, A&E rebroadcast Terri's interview with me.

Congress held hearings. Adding to the controversy, the chief investigator for the National Transportation Safety Board, the American agency charged with investigating air crashes, told the House Committee on Crime that he did not believe that ice caused the crash.

"It's a bloody cover-up," dissenting CASB member Roger Lacroix told the press. "Just about everybody who knows something about flying will say it's not ice." Anyone can make such a statement, but Lacroix had strong credentials. He was a retired brigadier general and a combat pilot with the Royal Canadian Mounted Police.[20]

"It's a major, major national cover-up and scandal, and it's documented," stated Gene Wheaton, a former agent with the US Army Criminal Investigation Division. "What you've got here is a criminal conspiracy between certain folks in the U.S. and certain folks in Canada to write a fraudulent report, and you've got another massive criminal conspiracy to cover up a probable mass murder—a terrorist act—and allowing the perpetrators to go free."[21]

More than one hundred members of Congress signed a letter asking then president George Herbert Walker Bush to reopen the investigation and to release to the public all files and reports regarding the crash. Their requests were completely ignored.

I'm definitely not an aviation crash expert. But I don't think you have to be to determine something went terribly wrong in the

Gander investigation. My guess is that the Reagan administration knew that any major investigation into the allegations that terrorists may have caused the crash would have exposed Oliver North and the entire Iran-Contra scandal. As a result, the US military and the administration were more than willing to just accept the Canadian report and move on.

To me, one of the most mysterious elements of this entire story involves those six crates that were placed in the cargo bay in Cairo. The best examination of this part of the case was done by Janet Crawley, a reporter who covered the White House for the *Chicago Tribune*. Crawley referred to the boxes as "wooden footlockers" that were "coffin-shaped." The boxes were six feet by two feet by fourteen inches.[22]

"The official version of the contents of the boxes is varied," Crawley wrote in an article published on April 22, 1990. "An Army spokesman said in a letter last fall that they contained 'passenger comfort kits,' which generally are defined as containing things like Handi Wipes and eating utensils."

The article then stated that the Defense Department provided Congress with a manifest showing that the boxes contained spare airplane parts. The CASB claimed that medical records were in the boxes. The article also cited other knowledgeable sources asserting there were either missiles in the boxes and antitank rockets or the bodies of US commandos who died in a secret attempt to free US hostages in Lebanon.[23]

Then there's a mystery regarding what happened to the boxes after the crash. The *Chicago Tribune*, a Republican-leaning newspaper not known for publishing wild-eyed conspiracies, quoted the president of the Union of Canadian Transport Employees, which included many of the firefighters and rescue workers in Gander, saying that US military officials "found five of the boxes" and quickly removed the crates from the crash site and aboard a US military plane "under cover of darkness."[24]

Terri Taylor told me she interviewed firefighters at the crash site who informed her that US military officials roped off the area where the boxes were found and prohibited rescue workers from getting anywhere close to them.

So what really happened to Arrow Air Flight 950?

Here's what I know for sure:

The Canadian Aviation Safety Board's majority report stated that there was no evidence of a fire onboard the plane prior to the crash. The CASB and the AFIP jointly agreed that the 248 soldiers and 8 crew members died instantaneously when the jetliner slammed into the ground.

The toxicology reports prove that this is simply untrue. More than fifty soldiers had carbon monoxide levels of 70 percent or higher. The only explanation is that they inhaled the deadly toxin while onboard the airplane prior to the crash and prior to their deaths.

The official investigation and conclusion is fatally flawed and totally in error.

The first President George Bush refused to reopen the Gander investigation. The second President Bush should correct the error of his father and do it now. I would think that in light of September 11, 2001, this administration and our government would want to be truthful to the American public about terrorist acts.

The American public deserves to know the truth about Arrow Air Flight 950. The families of all those soldiers who died deserve to know. If our government will not tell us the truth about this case, how can we trust them in the future?

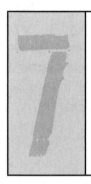

JANE BOLDING

ANGEL OF DEATH OR
VICTIM OF STATISTICS?

Just the phrases Angel of Mercy and Angel of Death conjure up all kinds of images and stereotypes, theories and beliefs. To some, an Angel of Mercy speaks of compassion and love, a kind and giving heart devoted to relieving pain and freeing the spirit. The Angel of Death, in contrast, is considered an evil agent that preys on the weak and elderly, and kills the defenseless.

The term Angel of Death has its roots in the biblical story when God was said to have sent an angel to Egypt to take the life of the firstborn son in every family in order to convince Pharaoh to release his Hebrew captives. Angel of Death was also the name later given to Josef Mengele, the evil Nazi physician who supervised the vicious experiments upon and execution of tens of thousands of Jews at a concentration camp in Auschwitz. For many the phrase brings to mind the picture of Dr. Jack Kevorkian hooking up suffering patients to his death machine. Moreover, there have been countless reports of hospital nurses and medical personnel accused of killing patients whom they are supposed to be treating.

I've always had a personal problem with the way the mainstream media seems to glorify the people identified as Angels of

175

Mercy or Angels of Death. Doctors and nurses take an oath to preserve and nurture life. They should not be glorified for actions in which they violate that oath or promise. I understand that these cases are newsworthy. The conflict of a healthcare giver taking a life is indeed fascinating. And I suspect that there are more instances of physicians, nurses, and other medical personnel taking steps to end a life in order to relieve pain and suffering than we could ever imagine. The National Legal Center for the Medically Dependent and Disabled reported in March 2003 that there have been eighteen people accused of "quiet killings" in US hospitals during the past twenty years. The center reported that a dozen of those individuals were convicted and sentenced to serve time in prison.[1]

These so-called Angels of Death are usually medical staff personnel, many of whom are taking these actions because—at least in their own minds—they believe they are Angels of Mercy, relieving the pain and suffering of someone who is critically ill and suffering severely, and who is near death anyway. They, in general, are not doing this in cases where a patient has come to the hospital to have an appendectomy or to have a bunion repaired.

One of the first of those alleged eighteen cases—and possibly the highest profile of the group—involved a Maryland nurse named Jane Bolding. The case surfaced in 1985 when the young nurse was arrested in conjunction with an investigation into the deaths of scores of patients at the hospital where she worked. The case made national newspaper headlines, was featured on the evening network newscasts, and was the subject of many magazine articles.

As a forensic pathologist hired as a medical expert in the case, I was given a front-row seat to the real-life drama. It was a case that took a number of twists and turns. There were many people who believed Bolding killed several of her patients. There were just as many individuals who were convinced she was completely innocent and had done nothing wrong.

The case of Jane Bolding taught me that the facts do not always add up to the truth. To best understand what truly happened, you must understand the sequence of events.

In 1985 Prince George's County Hospital was considered one of the nation's finest institutions of healing for the seriously ill in the United States. A regional trauma center in suburban Washington, DC, the 555-bed nonprofit hospital that was operated by county officials, served a four-county area. In 1985 the hospital averaged about 350 patients a day.

While the medical center was a full-service hospital with an emergency room, birthing facilities, and radiology, cardiology, and respiratory departments, the center's intensive care unit (ICU) was considered one of its gems. The ICU was a sixteen-bed unit designed to handle the most critically ill patients. The patients in the ICU required nearly constant care. Many were near death.

Because patients in intensive care have so many needs, additional staffing is required at any hospital that operates an ICU. At Prince George's County Hospital in 1985, three full-time and five part-time physicians attended to the intensive care patents. In addition, surgical and medical residents were also on regular ICU duty. Normally, there would be six to eight registered nurses also working the ICU during each of the hospital's three shifts.

There's no question that the hospital at that time was one of the best run medical centers on the East Coast. Its staff was unquestionably committed to the health and welfare of the public it served. But nothing prepared the administrators, doctors, nurses, and other hospital personnel for the firestorm that hit Prince George's County Hospital in March 1985.

During the first week of March, three medical personnel, including a nurse and a physician's assistant who worked in the intensive care unit, were talking among themselves, comparing notes. As they chatted, they remarked that there had been an unusual number of patients who had experienced cardiac arrests in the ICU over the previous few months.[2]

Just a coincidence? Probably, they all agreed. But each of them also commented on how nearly all of the attacks seemed to take place during one shift—the evening shift. Many of the cardiac arrests seemed to take place near the end of the evening shift, and a large number of the patients suffering the attacks seemed to be assigned to one bed—bed eight. And the trio noticed one other common denominator in the rash of incidents: one particular registered nurse always seemed to be on duty or attending to the patients who suffered cardiac arrest.

Jane Bolding.

Still just a coincidence? they wondered.

Maybe. Probably. Had to be.

After all, the three agreed that Jane Bolding, who was twenty-seven years old, was one of the most caring, attentive nurses in the ICU. The patients and their families loved Jane, and she appeared to truly care for them. The doctors, nurses, and other ICU staff members admired her passion for the job and her compassion for the sickest of the sick. The hospital and the ICU patients were her life, her devotion. The worst thing that could be said about Jane, they joked, was that she was disorganized.

Agreeing that they were probably wrong in their perceptions, the trio also felt an overriding need to share their suspicions with their supervisors. Hours later, their comments had circulated from the ICU supervisor to the chief of medicine and to the hospital administrators and lawyers. The rumor, even if completely unfounded, needed to be checked out.

After a brief review of medical records, hospital officials decided to conduct an internal inquiry.[3] The pathology reports on the patients who died showed larger than expected levels of potassium chloride in their bodies at the times of death. Potassium chloride is an electrolyte, or mineral, naturally found in the human body. But too much of it can cause cardiac arrest.

As part of the in-house probe, hospital authorities interviewed doctors and nurses who worked with Bolding. Few had anything bad to say about her. And none testified that she was acting suspiciously or that they had witnessed her do anything inappropriate. Nor was there any evidence that any potassium chloride was missing.

Jane Bolding was the last person asked to appear before the committee.[4] She clearly had no idea why she was being interviewed, what the review process was about, or that she was the focus of the inquiry, according to transcripts of the proceeding. The registered nurse appeared openly distraught when confronted with the idea that so many of her patients seemed to be dying. She displayed a genuine anguish over the death of each person, even crying at times when wondering aloud if there was not more she could have done to save each person's life.

Bolding's sincerity combined with her sterling record as a registered nurse left some on the committee confident that she had done nothing wrong. Even so, the panel agreed that Bolding should be placed on administrative leave with pay pending the outcome of its audit. Hospital officials told Bolding that there would be a meeting on the inquiry on March 19 at 4 PM. She was told that she should be present at that meeting to hear the committee's findings and recommendations. She would also have an opportunity to speak.

Initially, medical center officials wanted to keep their internal inquiry private. The last thing that hospital leaders wanted was for this suspicion to become public, especially if there was no truth to the notion that patients were dying under questionable circumstances. The medical center's administrators and physicians agreed that if the allegations were made public, it might cause a public health panic, scaring patients away from the hospital. They also knew it would certainly bring negative media attention to the hospital as well.

But the secrecy ended the second week of March when local police received an anonymous tip from a hospital employee. The confidential informant told police that there had been an extremely large number of deaths in the hospital's intensive care unit, that the hospital knew it, that it was conducting a secret internal inquiry, and that the hospital's investigation into the cause of the problem was focused on a specific nurse.[5]

Within hours, Prince George County's police chief was on the telephone with the hospital's general counsel and the physician in charge of the intensive care unit. The next day, homicide detectives were combing the medical facility for evidence, interviewing doctors, nurses, and technicians. They also seized the medical records of the patients who had died.

On the morning of March 19, two homicide detectives from Prince George's County Police Department knocked on Bolding's door at her home on Capitol Hill in southeast Washington, DC. The investigators asked if she would go with them to the police station to answer some questions about the situation at the hospital. Bolding spoke briefly with a lawyer for the hospital, who told her that it was appropriate for her to speak with the police to tell them what she knew. She agreed, but told the detectives that she needed to be at the hospital at 4 PM for the meeting with the administration.[6]

It was a meeting Jane Bolding would not attend.

At first, the detectives seemed friendly. They offered her coffee and Coca-Cola. They spent a couple hours having Bolding review her life and career as a nurse. Then they talked about individual patients, many of whom had died under her care. Some of the questions that the investigators asked included:

Was it difficult to watch the patients suffer day after day?

How did she feel when they died?

Had she ever thought about how the lives of these patients were in her hands?

Did she believe in God?

Did she think the patients were probably in heaven?

Had she suffered any personal losses of life or tragedies in her own family?

Bolding answered the questions as they were asked. She seemed confused at times about why she was being asked these types of questions. But she said she recognized that the detectives were just doing their jobs and she wanted to cooperate as much as she could.

All the while, Bolding's coffee cup was constantly refilled.

By midafternoon, the informational inquiry had become a full-blown interrogation. The attitude of the detectives had purportedly changed from being friendly and comforting to confrontational and combative. The questions had become harsh and much more pointed.

Did she think the patients were better off dead?

Was there a sense of relief or comfort when the patients died?

Did she sympathize with their suffering?

Would these patients have gotten better or ever been able to live normal lives?

Did she ever think that the extreme cost of treating intensive care patients who most likely would never recover was taking away resources from patients who could be helped?

Unbeknownst to Bolding, the hospital attorney who had told her it was okay to talk to the detectives showed up at the police station. But he was informed that she did not want to see a lawyer and he would not be permitted to talk to her. Bolding was never told that the lawyer was outside and wanted to speak with her.

Inside the interrogation room, Bolding was getting tired. She had answered so many questions. She wanted a break. She kept telling the detectives that she had two dogs at home that had been locked up in her house all day. They needed water and to be let outside. Instead, the investigators insisted they had only a few more questions. The caffeine kept being poured. As the afternoon became evening and then night, new detectives joined the interrogation. They asked many of the same questions over and over. The initial detectives were sent home to get some sleep. But Jane Bolding was forced to continue answering questions all night long.

She told detectives how her mother, during a heated argument, had blurted out that she had been adopted, a fact that the four-teen-year-old Jane had not known before. She told police that she had been physically abused as a young child and how she had been raped in 1980 outside of her apartment on Capitol Hill.[7]

For hours and hours, Bolding never wavered in her response. Of course she felt sorry for the terminally ill patients. Yes, they deserved to be free of their pain and suffering. Absolutely, the families of the ICU patients were suffering, too.

Through it all, Bolding categorically denied that she wished any ill will on any of the patients. She adamantly denied playing any role in their deaths. And she was unflinching in her statement that she had never, never injected any of the patients on the ICU ward with doses of potassium chloride that had not been prescribed by the attending physicians.

But as the sun rose on Prince George's County Police Department, Jane Bolding was tired. She cried and cried as detectives went over the files of each patient who had died during her watch.

"These people are dead and they died during your shift, while you were supposed to be watching over them," an investigator stated. "Don't you feel bad about that? Don't you feel bad that they died in your care?"[8]

Bolding, weakened by the deprivation of sleep and jittery from too much caffeine, cried some more, saying she was so sorry and felt horrible for their deaths. Finally, she uttered the words detectives had been waiting to pounce on. Bolding told them that, yes, she did feel responsible for the deaths.

"That's because you are responsible for their deaths, aren't you?" one detective stated from across the room. "It's okay. It feels good to get these feelings off your chest. It will help lift the guilt that you're feeling."[9]

The detectives, realizing they had Bolding on the verge of a confession, pushed harder. They told her that it was okay to admit that she felt the patients had suffered long enough. They said it was totally reasonable for her to want to end their pain. They said a lot of people wouldn't blame her for taking the steps necessary to alleviate the suffering of the patients.

After more than twenty-three hours of continuous interrogation, Bolding, in a state of complete exhaustion, admitted she had injected one of her patients, Elinor Dickerson, with a dose of potassium chloride. But the detectives weren't satisfied. They continued to push Bolding to confess more.

During the next eleven hours, they convinced Bolding to write a letter of apology to Mrs. Dickerson's son. A sixty-nine-year-old diabetic, Mrs. Dickerson had undergone coronary bypass surgery at Prince George's County Hospital. In September 1984 doctors had moved her to ICU following the surgery after she started bleeding in her esophagus. Physicians and nurses agreed that Dickerson was in a poor mental state and her health was declining.

In all, three different shifts of detectives interrogated Bolding nonstop for thirty-four hours. Based on Bolding's supposed confession letter, police charged her with first-degree murder in the death of Dickerson. The crime was punishable by a sentence of life in prison. The police notified the local medical examiner that Bolding had confessed to killing Dickerson. The hospital pathologist, who had listed Dickerson's cause of death as natural at the time she died, officially changed his determination to homicide.

That afternoon Bolding was transported from the police station to the county jail to be booked and to be held pending trial. As police led Bolding from the police station into the bright light of the sun, they were confronted by hordes of television cameras and news reporters shouting questions at the nurse and the detectives. The video of Bolding, suffering from exhaustion caused by two days witout sleep and the psychological and emotional drain of thirty-four hours of intense interrogation, was replayed time and again on the news.

I remember reading about Bolding's arrest in the *New York Times* and in the Pittsburgh newspapers. The articles cited police sources as saying that the nurse had confessed. Like everyone else who read those articles, I assumed that the case was open-and-shut. After all, most confessions are the result of one of two things: a guilty conscience or admission after being confronted with overwhelming evidence.

While the police, through the news media, asserted Bolding's guilt, the case quietly had problems from the start. The moment that the case file was turned over to the state attorney's office, prosecutors recognized major flaws in the evidence.

There was a question about whether police had told Bolding that she was a suspect and that she had the right to remain silent and the right to legal counsel, as required by the US Supreme Court in the *Miranda* case.[10] There also was the fact that a hospital lawyer had come to the police station to talk to Bolding as she was being interrogated but was told that Bolding did not want to talk to a lawyer—a statement that was less than true. And finally, there was the fact that detectives had interrogated Bolding for thirty-four consecutive hours. Thirty-four hours. My days in law school and as an assistant district attorney told me that thirty-four hours of police interrogation was going to create significant constitutional problems for the state.

Indeed, seven weeks later, Prince George's state attorney, Arthur "Bud" Marshall Jr., filed a court motion seeking to dismiss the murder charge against Bolding.[11] He cited the constitutional issues surrounding the interrogation of Bolding. But he promised to continue the investigation at the hospital.

A month later Bolding was back at the hospital's intensive care unit standing over a critically ill patient. This time security guards stood at her side. Sadly, this patient also died as Bolding looked on. But this patient was her father. He passed away convinced that his daughter was innocent and believing that her legal problems were behind her.

But the case was far from over.

Prosecutors told the detectives to start their investigation over. The police were instructed to reinterview the original witnesses at the hospital. New witnesses were identified and questioned. And the medical records were scoured in the search for new evidence.

Yet nothing new emerged. No one saw Bolding doing anything suspicious. No one witnessed her sneaking potassium chloride from the hospital's pharmacy or injecting any patients with unauthorized needles. No one came forward to testify that Bolding had confessed to them.

Feeling community pressure to solve the case, prosecutors turned for help to the federal Centers for Disease Control in Atlanta. The CDC, an agency of the US government that investigates trends in national health issues, initially declined to get involved. But prosecutors in Prince George's County enlisted the help of the US Justice Department to convince the CDC that the case needed its help.

By late November 1985 the CDC was on the job. A team of medical experts was put together by the CDC and gathered at Prince George's County Hospital for two days of meetings. Leading the team was Dr. Jeffrey J. Sacks, who was an epidemiologist for the CDC. The team was given copies of the medical records seized by police from the hospital. The ICU's hospital staff told them about their procedures and practices regarding the administration of medicine.

On December 5 the CDC experts flew home to Atlanta to analyze their data. The CDC studied thousands of medical records and charts from each patient who had been admitted to Prince George's County Hospital in 1983, 1984, and 1985. The group identified patient demographics and trends with the goal of determining whether an epidemic of cardiac arrests or deaths had occurred at the hospital. The cases were examined to see when the events had occurred, what were the causes of the attacks, and who were the staff on duty at the time the cardiac arrests took place. Thanks to detailed logs in the hospital's ICU, the researchers were even able to identify specific beds in the unit where the deaths took place.

On July 14, 1986, Dr. Sacks issued the CDC's findings in a nineteen-page report that included an additional fifteen pages of charts and graphics. The report began:

An epidemic of cardiac arrests occurred in a Prince George's County Hospital intensive care unit from January 1984—March 1985. The records of 93 percent of all admissions from 1983 to 1985 were reviewed and verified to characterize the epidemic. The cardiac arrests occurred predominantly during the last four hours of the evening shift. The most significant risk factor for a cardiac arrest was having a specific nurse as the attendant."[12]

The report identified that person as "Nurse 14."

Nurse 14 was not identified in the report. But it was clear to all who knew anything about the investigation that it referred to Jane Bolding.

The CDC study found that Bolding was the nurse attending to 57 of the 144 (40 percent) cardiac arrests that occurred in the ICU during the fifteen months examined. The next highest number of cardiac arrests connected to a specific nurse was five, or only 3 percent of the cases. The finger was pointed even more strongly at Bolding when the report stated that 65 percent of the eighty-eight cardiac arrests during the evening shift were patients of Nurse 14.

"One bed, the least visible from the nursing station, was the location of a disproportionate share of the evening shift and Nurse 14's cardiac arrest patients," according to the study. "Upon admission to the ICU, cardiac arrest patients attended by Nurse 14 had similar prognoses and admitting conditions as did patients attended by other nurses. Nurse 14's cardiac arrest patients were more likely to have unexplained elevations of potassium and did not fit the typical profile of a PGH [Prince George's Hospital] ICU arrest patient. They were young, more often female, and had had recent surgery."[13]

The CDC report also found that ICU patients were four times more likely to have cardiac arrests when Bolding was on duty than when she was not on duty. And Bolding's patients were thirty-five to ninety-six times more likely to experience cardiac arrest than the patients of other ICU nurses.

"The epidemic, as well as the unusual time, place, and person clustering, ceased when Nurse 14 was no longer employed in the ICU," concluded Dr. Sacks, the author of the examination.[14]

By fall 1986, law enforcement officials in Prince George's County had become frustrated with their inquiry into Bolding. No new evidence had been uncovered. No smoking gun, so to speak, had ever surfaced. But in November the CDC turned its findings over to prosecutors. The report completely reinvigorated the investigation.

Prosecutors and police met with the medical examiner to review the files of the patients who had suffered cardiac arrests under Bolding's care. The patients who showed the most significant increases in the level of potassium were given the highest priority. Detectives then reinterviewed the families of those patients.

In mid-December prosecutors and police felt they had collected enough evidence once again to charge Bolding for some of the deaths at the hospital. However, prosecutors decided against sending officers to the nurse's home to arrest her. Instead, authorities, realizing the case would be very high profile, chose to present their evidence—new and old—to the local state grand jury and to ask that panel officially to charge Bolding by issuing an indictment.

State grand juries are usually comprised of twelve to eighteen local citizens who serve anywhere from six weeks to eighteen months. Grand jury proceedings are completely secret. Only one side—the prosecution—gets to present evidence and its argument. The grand jurors and the prosecutors are prohibited by law from discussing anything that goes on inside the grand jury room. Only witnesses who testify before the grand jury are permitted to talk publicly about what questions they were asked and their answers. Unlike jurors, grand jurors are permitted to ask questions of the witnesses and the prosecutors.

After the evidence has been presented, the grand jurors vote on whether they believe there is sufficient evidence for the case to proceed to trial. While juries are required to find a defendant guilty "beyond a reasonable doubt," grand jurors only have to determine that there is "probable cause" to believe that the defendant committed the crime. If the grand jury finds that there is not enough evidence to find "probable cause," the panel can refuse to issue an indictment. If the grand jury does issue an indictment, the defendant is then required to stand trial on the charges listed in the indictment. But it also requires that the prosecutors prove that the charges listed in the indictment are true.

On December 16, 1986, Assistant State's Attorney Jay Creech presented the new case to the Prince George's County grand jury. The panel heard about the deaths at the hospital. They were told about the high levels of potassium detected in the autopsies of the patients. They were shown the CDC study and its findings. They were told about Bolding's confession to the police and the letter she wrote to Dickerson's family.

The grand jurors, after reviewing the evidence, found that probable cause existed to charge Bolding. The indictment they issued that day accused Bolding of killing three patients in her ICU ward and attempting to kill two other patients. The indictment named the five patients Bolding allegedly tried to kill. They were:

- Elinor Dickerson, the sixty-nine-year-old diabetic Bolding was initially charged with murdering. She died in September 1984 after undergoing coronary bypass surgery.
- Martha Moore, a forty-four-year-old friend of Bolding, who was admitted to the ICU after her lungs and kidneys failed. She died in October 1984.
- Isadore Shreiber, a sixty-nine-year-old who died in October 1984 after suffering from respiratory failure and poorly functioning kidneys.
- Gordon Dobson, a sixteen-year-old who was admitted to the hospital after suffering a severe head injury and major

internal trauma to several organs in a car accident. He suffered six cardiac arrests over a three-day period in March 1985. However, he did not die.

- Mary Mortbeto, a thirty-eight-year-old who was being treated for severe bacterial pneumonia and respiratory failure. She suffered cardiac arrest in February 1984, but did not die.

Hours after the grand jury issued an indictment, police took Bolding into custody and officially charged her with the three homicides and the two attempted murders.

I was officially contacted by Burt Kahn, one of Bolding's lawyers, in the spring of 1987. Kahn needed a forensic expert to examine the state's evidence and possibly testify at the trial. When they approached me, however, the lawyers said they had a problem. Their representation of Bolding was court appointed, meaning they were being paid only a minimal amount by the state for their time. In addition, the state of Maryland would allow them to spend very little money to hire independent experts.

The bottom line was they had no money to pay me. Even so, I found the facts in the case so fascinating that I told Burt Kahn that I would assist in their case on a pro bono basis. The state would merely have to pay for my travel expenses.

As part of their investigation, prosecutors and the Prince George's County medical examiner had exhumed the body of Mrs. Dickerson in 1985 to conduct a second autopsy. Now authorities announced they were going to exhume the bodies of Martha Moore and Isadore Shreiber in order to conduct second autopsies on each. Bolding's lawyers asked me to attend. I agreed.

The exhumations and autopsies were scheduled for May 15, 1987. Four days prior to my flying to Baltimore to observe the exhumations and autopsies, I received in the mail from Bolding's lawyers a copy of the earlier exhumation autopsy in the Mrs. Dickerson case and a copy of the original death certificates in the

Moore and Shreiber cases. The package also included twenty-two sets of medical records involving other alleged victims at Prince George's County Hospital. These were medical records that were seized by the police and were still being investigated, although no charges had been filed regarding them. But it was the three death cases—Dickerson, Moore, and Shreiber—that I was instructed to focus on.

Name: Elinor S. Dickerson
Date of Death: 09/29/84
Place of Death: Prince George's County Hospital
Hour: 12:05 AM
Sex: Female
Race: White
Height: four feet eleven inches
Weight: 127 lbs
Date of Birth: January 13, 1915
Place of Birth: Beaverdam, Virginia
Marriage Status: Widowed
Occupation: Housewife
Immediate Cause of Death: Cardiac Arrest due to internal bleeding, infection, pneumonia
Place of Burial: Ebenezer Methodist Church Cemetery in Garrisonville, Virginia

According to documents filed by the State of Maryland Department of Post Mortem Examiners, Dickerson's body was exhumed on April 12, 1985. However, the second autopsy was not performed until six days later. The autopsy was handled by the state's chief medical examiner with officials from Prince George's County present.

The "Examination Record" reported the following:

The body of an embalmed, exhumed white female is received. The body and clothing are very moist. The skin of the hands is somewhat wrinkled from moisture. The hair is 5" long and gray.

The body is clothed in a blue lacy nightgown/robe. There is a blue silk nightie under this and a slip. The skin of the feet is sloughing from the moisture. The eye color is obscured from the embalming procedure. Pink lipstick remains. The jaws are wired closed.

The autopsy went on to describe the scars that appear as a result of the initial hospital postmortem examination and the subsequent embalming by the funeral home prior to burial. The report portrayed Mrs. Dickerson as a sixty-nine-year-old diabetic with arteriosclerotic heart disease. She was in postoperative surgery for extensive bleeding in her esophagus when she suffered a cardiac arrest. This second autopsy attributed it to a sudden increase in serum potassium levels.

My initial thought was that there was nothing in either the first or the second autopsy that raised my suspicion of foul play. Hospital records did show that Mrs. Dickerson's potassium levels were dangerously high. Indeed, her potassium rose from 3.2 several hours before her cardiac arrest to 7.8 when she suffered the arrest at midnight. But it was totally unclear to me that the high potassium levels were the primary contributor to her death. After all, Mrs. Dickerson was a very sick woman. Her body was weak and ravaged by diabetes and heart disease. But even if potassium played a role in her death, there was absolutely no evidence in the autopsy that the potassium was improperly injected into her body.

The second file I examined on my plane trip was that of Isadore Shreiber, a sixty-nine-year-old man who died in the ICU at Prince George's County Hospital about two weeks after Mrs. Dickerson's death. His original autopsy report read as follows:

Name: Isadore Shreiber
Date of Death: 10/12/84
Hour of Death: 7:50 PM
Place of Death: Prince George's County Hospital
Sex: Male

Race: Caucasian
Date of Birth: November 2, 1914
Place of Birth: Pennsylvania
Marital Status: Married
Occupation: Bus Driver
Weight: 173 lbs
Height: five feet eleven inches
Cause of Death: Cardiopulmonary Arrest

According to the hospital reports, Mr. Shreiber was hospitalized on September 10, complaining that his feet had been swelling and his toes had been turning blue during the summer months. His medical history included diabetes, hypertension, and three myocardial infarcts (heart attacks). Ten days after Mr. Shreiber was hospitalized, he experienced an acute shortness of breath, diagnosed as congestive heart failure. He also exhibited signs of severe infection and deterioration of the respiratory system. He suffered a respiratory arrest on October 3 and cardiac arrest on October 12. He did not survive the latter.

The original autopsy, performed by a pathologist at Prince George's County Hospital on November 15, 1984, declared the cause of death to be a cardiac arrest combined with acute renal failure. The autopsy found nothing that raised any suspicion. But internal hospital records showed that Mr. Shreiber's potassium levels were dramatically increased at the time he experienced the cardiac arrest that took his life.

The third death case under review was that of Martha Moore, whose body we were scheduled to exhume that afternoon. Information from the initial autopsy performed by hospital pathologists was included in the file.

Name: Martha G. Moore
Date of Death: 10/28/84
Hour: 5:40 PM
Place of Death: Prince George's County Hospital

Sex: Female
Race: Black
Date of Birth: May 7, 1940
Place of Birth: Brandywine, Maryland
Marriage Status: Never Married
Occupation: Receptionist at Prince George's County Hospital
Cause of Death: Cardiac Pulmonary Arrest

The original autopsy was also performed by a hospital pathologist a few hours after Ms. Moore died. The autopsy concluded that
a cardiopulmonary attack combined with renal failure and symp-
toms associated with sarcoidosis, a disease characterized by small
lesions on internal organs or tissue, contributed to the death.

My flight from Pittsburgh to Baltimore-Washington International Airport took less than forty minutes. But it was during that
time that Maryland officials decided to postpone the exhumation
of Mr. Shreiber until a later date.

I arrived just as Ms. Moore's body was being exhumed from the
Asbury Cemetery in Brandywine, Maryland. It was transported by
ambulance to the office of the Maryland chief medical examiner in
Baltimore. Martha Moore's casket was brought in first at about
10:05 AM. The casket had been sealed since burial. The corpse was
wrapped in a full-length plastic body bag that had a zipper in the
front. The body was dressed in a white billowy gown. Underneath,
she wore a brown slip, beige brassiere, pale blue underwear, and
pantyhose with plastic coverings. A white hospital bracelet on the
left ankle bore the name of the deceased.

A photographer for the medical examiner's office snapped pictures every few seconds from all different angles.

Once the clothes were removed, the examination began. The
body had been embalmed and remained in good condition. The
skin had begun to deteriorate in the neck, arms, and legs. Her eyes
were sunken and her black scalp hair was medium in length. The
mouth was fixed in a closed position. The nails on her fingers were

covered with red polish. However, some of the nails slipped off as the body was repositioned on the examination table. The fingers and toes exhibited significant mummification.

The body's midsection exhibited a twelve-inch sutured incision and the Y-shaped incision at the chest plate that was done during the initial autopsy. The body cavities were examined, but there was no evidence of injury. The partial removal of the skull also detected no signs of foul play.

For more than two hours, we reexamined every aspect of Ms. Moore's body, as if we were performing the autopsy for the first time. We inspected the neck and face. We examined the heart, lungs, liver, and kidneys.

At age forty-four, Ms. Moore and her body showed evidence of a prolonged struggle with sarcoidosis, the lung disease that requires extensive steroid treatment. Our autopsy revealed signs of advanced heart disease with significant areas of scarring to the heart tissue—the likely result of the sarcoidosis and the steroid therapy. The hospital's physicians had noted in her medical chart that she had a "poor prognosis for survival."

Ms. Moore had been treated for failure of the kidney filtration system to function. She also had undergone surgery to repair a perforation of the small intestine and subsequent infection of the abdominal cavity. And just prior to her death, she suffered an acute renal failure that required dialysis.

The original autopsy report filed by hospital pathologists at the time of Ms. Moore's death included ICU records from Prince George's County Hospital showing that the patient's potassium levels took an unexpected increase—from 5.1 to 10.4—on the evening she suffered the cardiac arrest and died. However, the second autopsy showed no evidence that potassium had been injected into her system.

The case languished for several months in a sort of procedural holding pattern. There were scores of court hearings to debate admissibility of evidence. There were fights over the CDC report and whether it could be introduced as evidence at trial or whether it should be excluded. There were battles over the reliability of medical records taken from the hospital. But most important, there were lengthy hearings and multiple briefs filed by both sides over the admissibility of Jane Bolding's statements to police, as well as the alleged confession or apology letter she wrote to Mrs. Dickerson's family.

On January 18, 1988, the state's case seemed to be bolstered when Maryland Chief Medical Examiner Dr. John E. Smialek issued his long-awaited official opinion on the deaths of Dickerson, Moore, and Shreiber. Dr. Smialek, a respected forensic pathologist, said that he had "reviewed the medical records regarding the treatment of Elinor Dickerson in the Prince George's County Hospital prior to her death on September 29, 1984; information provided to [him] by Prince George's County Police Department related to the investigation of this death; and clinical assessments of Mrs. Dickerson's clinical status prior to her death by outside experts."

Dr. Smialek concluded:

> Following my review of this information, it is my opinion that Mrs. Dickerson died as the result of non-therapeutic administration of potassium into the intravenous tubing while she was a patient in the Prince George's County Hospital and was being treated for severe therosclerotic cardiac vascular disease for which she had undergone a triple bypass graft.
> The manner of death is HOMICIDE.

However, Dr. Smialek was less confident in the opinions he issued in the Moore and Shreiber cases. In each, he declared the manner of death "undetermined." But he stated in both that he "cannot rule out the possibility of the non-therapeutic administration of potassium."

I was stunned the first time I read Dr. Smialek's official findings. First, I felt his opinion that Mrs. Dickerson was murdered was completely unsubstantiated by the medical evidence. I had reviewed the same autopsy report that Dr. Smialek had. I had read the same hospital records that he had. There was, quite simply, no scientific medical evidence that came anywhere close to showing that Mrs. Dickerson had been murdered. The autopsy had revealed nothing.

Mrs. Dickerson was a very sick woman. She was an insulin-dependent diabetic. She experienced severe bleeding in the esophagus. She had a history of coronary artery bypass surgery and had previously tested positive for Hepatitis A. Her blood sugar was extremely elevated, while her mental state was severely depressed. The medical evidence revealed that any number of Mrs. Dickerson's ailments could have caused or contributed significantly to her cardiac arrest.

Second, while I completely agree with Dr. Smialek's final conclusion in the Moore and Shreiber cases that the manner of their death was undetermined, I was astonished by his opinion that he "cannot rule out" the possibility that Ms. Moore and Mr. Shreiber were illegally injected with potassium with the intent to kill them.

Dr. Smialek seemed to be saying that he believed the state's case, even though he could find no evidence to support it. He also could have included that he found no evidence linking these two deaths to the assassination of President Kennedy or to an invasion of illegal aliens from outer space. Medical examiners conduct autopsies to uncover facts and determine truth. Autopsy findings are not about speculation or what *might* have happened. Autopsy reports are supposed to state one thing: medical evidence. Forensic pathology is a science.

The truth about the deaths of Ms. Moore and Mr. Shreiber is similar to that of Mrs. Dickerson. All three were extremely sick people, hence the reason they were patients in the intensive care unit of the hospital. By mere definition, these three patients were so ill, so fragile, so near death that they each required intensive medical attention twenty-four hours a day.

Ms. Moore's heart, lungs, liver, and kidneys, according to the autopsy and her medical records, were devastated by the sarcoidosis. Mr. Shreiber's body was in even worse shape, according to the reports. Both individuals were on dialysis for renal insufficiency. Both were being intravenously fed hypertonic solutions with high glucose content to treat malnutrition. All three suffered from respiratory distress syndrome.

The medical charts and autopsies of all three tell one story: these were very sick people who were on the verge of dying.

The medical records clearly show that the three experienced significant increases in their potassium levels at the time when they suffered their cardiac arrests. The police, prosecutors, hospital physicians, and Dr. Smialek interpreted this to mean that the increased potassium levels caused the attacks.

However, there is an equally plausible theory. The severe and deteriorating medical conditions that each suffered could have triggered internal physiological changes that, in turn, caused the body to generate an increased level of potassium. In fact, there is just as much likelihood that the potassium increase was caused by other factors, such as the steroid treatments or the high fever. The fact is that the cardiac arrests could have contributed to the potassium levels increasing.

When the heart stops, oxygen is no longer distributed through the bloodstream. That causes the tissues and cells to break down, which causes stored up potassium to be released.

Upon reviewing Dr. Smialek's findings as well as all the autopsy and medical records, I informed Bolding's lawyers that I was prepared to testify that there is no way that anyone can say, to any degree of medical certainty, that these patients died from overdoses of potassium. The evidence quite simply does not support such a claim.

In late January 1988, the Bolding case took another turn. This time, it was in Bolding's favor.

In the weeks following the grand jury's indictment of Bolding, her defense lawyers had filed court motions seeking to have the alleged confession and the letter to Mrs. Dickerson's son excluded from the trial on the grounds that the extended interrogation had violated their client's Fifth Amendment right against self-incrimination. The lawyers argued that, while the statement wasn't a confession at all, any statement police obtained from Bolding after twenty-three hours of questioning violated her constitutional rights.

Defense attorney Fred Joseph, a prominent Maryland criminal defense attorney appointed by the state to represent Bolding, told Judge Casula that he remembered receiving a telephone call at his office on March 20, 1985, at 11:00 AM. The caller was a representative from the nurse's union. The caller stated that one of their members, Jane Bolding, had been taken into custody by police the night before, had been questioned all night long, and that no one was being allowed to see or talk to her.

"I was outraged and disgusted," Joseph told the judge. "The police convinced themselves that they had the right person and they convinced themselves that they had to extract a confession, and by God, they were going to get it no matter what they had to do."[15]

"They trampled on the rights of a citizen," he said.

To me, this was an easy decision for the court. It may have been two decades since I finished law school, but it was clear to me and everyone else that Prince George's police had stepped way over the line. The US Supreme Court grants police a lot of discretion in their efforts to convince suspects to confess. Detectives may attempt to trick defendants into making a confession or even lie to them. Law enforcement is allowed to tell suspects that they have incriminating evidence that simply does not exist. That being said, the Supreme Court and the lower courts have stated repeatedly that confessions must be voluntarily given, free of any physical or psychological coercion.

People are always telling me that they would never confess to a crime that they did not commit. People may think they would never incriminate themselves if they are innocent, but science and history say otherwise. During the Korean War, three dozen American airmen confessed to committing war crimes that they had nothing to do with. The tool used by the Communist interrogators to obtain the false confessions was extensive sleep deprivation. And these were military officers, young, healthy, and trained to handle such situations.[16]

What chance did Jane Bolding have?

On January 25, 1988, Maryland Circuit Judge Joseph Casula agreed, throwing out any statements Bolding had made to the police during the interrogation. "There are simply no short-cuts around the Constitution," the judge courageously ruled.

It would have been very easy for Judge Casula to pass the buck, so to speak, by allowing the confession to be presented during the trial and letting the appeals courts make the tough and controversial decision. But he didn't. The decision was politically unpopular, but it was also the law. I was very impressed by Judge Casula's handling of this case.

Obviously, so were the lawyers representing Jane Bolding. A few weeks after Judge Casula made his ruling that threw out the supposed confession, Mr. Joseph and Mr. Kahn, who were law partners, announced that they were waiving their client's right to a jury trial. Instead, they decided they would leave the question of Bolding's guilt or innocence up to Judge Casula.

There were two primary reasons the lawyers chose a bench trial instead of a jury trial. First, the case had gotten an enormous amount of publicity through the news media. This would have been a huge story anywhere. But this case happened to take place in a suburb of Washington, DC, where the *Washington Post* was the local newspaper. The *Post*'s coverage of the case had been extensive, but fair. It had reported on every detail—from Bolding's arrest and alleged confession to the CDC report and Judge Casula's decision to throw out Bolding's statement as inadmissible under the Fifth Amendment.

Many newspapers and television networks tend to be very biased in favor of law enforcement. They favor law enforcement because police officers and prosecutors tend to be their sources and they are also standing up for the rights of victims by arresting the bad guys. Therefore, many journalists unfortunately state that judges throw out confessions or dismiss charges against suspects based on "legal technicalities." I've never understood why journalists call violations of the US Constitution "technicalities." The Fourth Amendment right protecting us against illegal searches and seizures by the government and the Fifth Amendment right protecting people from being forced to make confessions are not "technicalities."

To the tremendous credit of the *Washington Post*, its reporters never criticized Judge Casula for his ruling that disallowed Bolding's statement as evidence. In fact, the paper did an excellent series of articles about how Prince George's police department needed reforms and cited the Bolding case as an example.

That being said, the *Post* and other media outlets had publicized the fact that Bolding had made a statement, which the police and prosecutors called a confession. Even though the judge would not allow the statement or any reference to it to be made during the trial, the statement had become public knowledge. Everyone knew about it. There's no doubt that the statement would be brought up during jury deliberations.

Don't get me wrong: I'm a huge believer in the jury system. Ninety-nine times out of one hundred, I would pick a jury to decide my case over a single judge. But juries are always risky, even when you have a convincing case. You never know how emotion is going to play a role in the jury's decision making. In the Bolding case, the supposed confession was just too big of a risk. Even though it was not admissible evidence, everyone knew about it, and there was a fear that the public knowledge of the alleged confession had tainted the jury pool.

The second reason the defense lawyers gave was the fact that Judge Casula's reputation as a fair and honest jurist was widely known. When he threw out Bolding's statement, the defense lawyers believed that he would give their client a fair trial. So they decided to roll the dice and waived their right to a trial by jury, as provided for in the Sixth Amendment of the US Constitution. Instead, they agreed to let Judge Casula decide the case.

Two months later, Bolding's defense team scored another significant victory. Dr. Smialek, the chief medical examiner, announced that he was changing his official opinion regarding manner of death in the Dickerson case from "homicide" to "undetermined." Dr. Smialek had based his initial determination on Bolding's alleged confession. With her statement no longer valid or admissible, Dr. Smialek decided to change his opinion, too. It was the right thing for Dr. Smialek to do.

However, it sent the state's case against Bolding spinning into uncertainty. The prosecution's own top medical witness would no longer testify that any of the deceased died from unnatural causes.

When the trial commenced on May 18, Assistant State Attorney Jay Creech admitted that his case would not be easy to prove. He portrayed Jane Bolding as an evil Angel of Death who, in the shadows of hospital corners, played God with the lives of her patients.

"For that reason, it should be of no surprise that the state cannot produce one witness who can say they saw Jane Bolding stick a syringe into the victims," Creech told Judge Casula. "Everyone thought that Jane Bolding was a good, competent nurse, full of compassion. There may have been saints in that unit, but there was a killer angel in their midst."[17]

I always felt Creech was being put in an awkward position and that he knew he was in the middle of a trial that he could not win. But the case was so big and so political that the thought of dismissing the charges against Bolding would have been unacceptable. Despite the lack of direct physical, scientific evidence, Creech did a very good job of organizing his case and presenting the evidence he did have.

Prosecutors opened their case by introducing the hospital's

medical records of each patient. Hospital personnel and physicians were called to testify about why they had been alerted to the extraordinary large number of cardiac arrests in the ICU.

Bolding's nursing supervisor, Helen Bradley, told the judge that Jane frequently asked to be assigned to the sickest patients in their ward. Bradley testified that potassium chloride was a drug that was always in supply in the ICU and that it was administered frequently to patients at the direction of the attending physicians. She also stated that up to thirty other people, including nurses and other hospital personnel, had daily contact with the patients.[18]

Prosecutors also tried to establish Bolding's mind-set as an Angel of Death through the testimony of two family members of those who died. The first witness was Mary Higgs, Martha Moore's twin sister, who said that Bolding told her that Moore's death was "inevitable." Higgs did admit under oath that she was a plaintiff in a multimillion-dollar civil lawsuit against Bolding and the hospital.[19]

The daughter of Mr. Shreiber, Sharon Hayes, told the judge that Nurse Bolding approached her after doctors talked to her about whether to take extreme medical measures to keep the patient alive, if he experienced a cardiac or respiratory attack. "She said, 'Maybe you won't have to make that decision,'" Hayes testified. She also stated that Bolding discouraged the family from having an autopsy performed.[20]

Under cross-examination, however, Hayes and Higgs testified that Bolding was the kindest, most caring, and most compassionate nurse in the intensive care unit.

Because Dr. Smialek had changed his official opinion in the Dickerson case from "homicide" to "undetermined," prosecutors felt they needed additional expert testimony to support their theory. One of the key forensic experts they called to the witness stand was my good friend Dr. Michael Baden, the former chief medical examiner of New York City.

The night before Michael was scheduled to testify, I spent several hours on the telephone discussing the medical records and the autopsy reports with the defense attorneys. I walked them through my findings, and I provided them with key questions to ask the state's witnesses. Part of my job was to make sure the lawyers were prepared to seize upon any opportunities that proved our side of the case.

As I've stated repeatedly, Michael is one of my best friends and he's an excellent forensic pathologist. But in this case, I believe that he was simply wrong. Michael told the judge that his review of the medical records and autopsies in each of the three deaths led him to believe that each one died as the result of potassium injected into their bodies. While I disagreed with Michael's testimony, he is a very good witness, and I think his testimony was the strongest evidence that the state introduced throughout the entire trial.

"There is no innocent explanation for the rise in the potassium to occur," Baden told the judge. "It had to come from someone administering it."[21]

One of the final witnesses called to testify was Dr. Jeffrey J. Sacks, the scientist at the federal Centers for Disease Control who led the hospital statistical study. Dr. Sacks took the witness stand the first week of June and testified first on direct examination and then under cross-examination for several days. Prosecutors clearly felt he was their star witness. The courtroom was packed with newspaper, magazine, and television journalists waiting to hear his testimony.

Truthfully, I wanted to hear what he had to say, too.

In a very low-key tone, Dr. Sacks walked the judge through his role in the study—how he initially got involved, how he reviewed the records, who was involved, and finally how they came to the conclusions they did. He indicated from the start that he didn't want to investigate this matter at all. He became involved only after the CDC received pressure from the US Department of Justice. But Dr. Sacks also admitted that he found the project fascinating and was now glad he had been assigned to the matter. The study had cost $250,000 to conduct, $16,000 of which was paid by Prince George's County.

Dr. Sacks told Judge Casula that Jane Bolding was the nurse for eighty-eight ICU patients at Prince George's County Hospital who had experienced cardiac arrests during the fifteen months he studied—many times more than any other nurse in the medical center's intensive care unit. The CDC scientist stated that health statistics projections show that only thirty-one cardiac arrests should have occurred during that time period on Nurse Bolding's watch.

"The chances of that happening by chance is about 1 in 100 trillion," he said. "It would be like picking out one second from all of time."[22]

Dr. Sacks testified that there was an average of 7.2 cardiac arrests each month in the ICU at the Prince George's Hospital while Bolding worked there. That figure dropped to 3.2 per month after Bolding left the hospital.

Under cross-examination by Kahn, Dr. Sacks readily admitted that his study had flaws. He said that while the numbers show that "Nurse 14" was the overwhelming common denominator in the deaths, the study in no way addresses intent. In addition, Dr. Sacks acknowledged that only doctors and nurses were included in his study. Other medical personnel, from physician assistants to hospital chaplains, were excluded because there was no record of their individual patient visits.

On the morning of Wednesday, June 15, prosecutors rested their case after calling twenty-eight witnesses to testify.[23]

Following a break for lunch, lawyers for Bolding presented Judge Casula with a motion for directed verdict. The motion, defense attorney Fred Joseph argued, sought to have the charges against their client dismissed because of a lack of evidence. He told the judge that the state, quite simply, had not met its burden of proving beyond a reasonable doubt that Bolding killed these patients intentionally.

Joseph said that there were no eyewitnesses linking Bolding to the crime. There were no fingerprints. No weapon was ever located. In fact, the medical examiner had declined to even declare any of these cases homicides.

"I've never gotten to the end of a murder case where the words 'homicide' or 'murder' were not uttered in the courtroom," Joseph said. "Despite all the charts, despite all the fancy footwork, we're still left with speculation."

Burt Kahn, whose legal specialty is medicine and science, told the judge that the CDC study proved nothing and had many flaws.

"Jane Bolding was the best nurse, the most skilled nurse, so she took care of the sickest patients in the intensive care unit," Kahn stated. "She took care of the sickest of the sick. They died because they were gravely ill."

Judge Casula asked prosecutors if they wanted to respond.

"The rapid rise in potassium is the key," Creech told the judge. He then recited the litany of statistics provided by Dr. Sacks as part of the CDC study, including the 1-in-100 trillion chance that all these patients died on Bolding's watch.

"Is that just some amazing coincidence?" Creech asked Judge Casula.

"Mere presence at the scene of a crime is not enough," the judge responded. "What criminal act on her part? Give me some little act, something she did, something that says she was the person who administered the potassium."

Judge Casula told the lawyers that he needed time to review the evidence and would announce his decision in a few days. If the judge denied the defense's motion, that would not have been the end of the trial. The defense would then have been allowed to put on its side of the case. I was told by Burt Kahn to be prepared to testify as possibly the first witness in the case.

Do statistics prove that these individuals were murdered? And more important, do they prove that Jane Bolding committed the murders if indeed they were murders? First, I think that these statistics were, by definition, probabilities. And probability is, also by definition, reasonable doubt.

Never before, nor ever since, has a homicide case proceeded to trial on an epidemiological study. There was no confession. There were no eyewitnesses. There was no physical, medical, or scientific evidence pointing to Jane Bolding as a killer.

On June 20, Judge Casula announced his ruling from the bench in open court. "The state at most has placed Bolding at the scene of the offenses. But that is insufficient to sustain a conviction. The state's reach hopelessly exceeded its grasp," Judge Casula ruled. "Simply put, the evidence failed to supply the missing link that would connect the defendant with alleged criminal acts."[24]

"A conviction cannot rest solely on a statistical study," he said. "It would create a mathematical quagmire."

Judge Casula then turned his attention directly to Jane Bolding, who sat in tears beside her lawyers. "You've suffered a lot of humiliation and embarrassment and anxiety," he said. "The criminal justice system is not perfect."

Case dismissed.

Jane Bolding was free to go.

Justice was served.

In 2004 I spoke with Burt Kahn, who continues to be one of the best and brightest trial lawyers in Maryland and Washington, DC. He told me that he, too, is convinced that Bolding was completely innocent of the charges. He and I agree that there was no evidence that any crimes actually had been committed.

Jane, he told me, moved south, where she went to work for a health insurance firm, processing and coding claims. He said she had worked her way up to management and was doing very well.

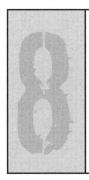

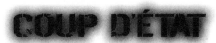

THE ASSASSINATION OF PRESIDENT JOHN F. KENNEDY

Washington, DC, can be very warm and muggy in late summer. The morning of August 24, 1972, was no different. I had flown from Pittsburgh to our nation's capital the afternoon before, had dinner that evening with friends and colleagues, and then returned to my hotel room for a solid night's sleep.

My wake-up call arrived at 6:30 AM. I showered, dressed, retrieved that morning's *Washington Post* at the foot of my door, and headed down to the café for coffee, orange juice, and a bagel. About 8 AM, the doorman flagged me a taxi.

"The National Archives, please."

Several blocks and three dollars later, I stood on the sidewalk in front of the prestigious National Archives Building. The massive concrete structure was quite intimidating. I walked to the main entrance and asked security to point me to Marion Johnson, the archivist who I was told would be expecting me.

In less than a minute, Mr. Johnson appeared. An affable man, he shook my hand and told me he was there to help me in any way he could. He led me to a large private room, which was nearly bare except for a table, a chair, an x-ray viewing machine, and a projector. There was no microscope available for me to use, so I had brought my own.

"Here's a list of the inventory," Mr. Johnson stated. "Let me know what you want to see and I will bring it to you for your inspection."

As I glanced down the multipage inventory, it was still hard to believe I was really here. After more than a year of requests, letter writing, phone calls, and in-person pleas, I was finally at the National Archives. I was about to examine the actual physical and medical evidence in the assassination of President John F. Kennedy. In doing so, I would become the first nongovernmental forensic pathologist to have official access to the evidence for purposes of scientific examination.

In 1965 federal officials, in their divine wisdom, chose to turn over all the physical evidence and autopsy materials to Jackie Kennedy. This was totally unheard of even in 1965 and remains absolutely unacceptable today. This was evidence in a crime. Authorities never turn over physical evidence and autopsy materials to the family. The fact that this was evidence in the assassination of our president makes the decision even more horrific.

In 1966 Mrs. Kennedy announced she was donating the materials to the National Archives. There was a caveat, however: the materials were not to be made public until after the death of her children. Nonetheless, she did say that recognized experts in the field of pathology would be allowed to apply to review the materials for "serious historical purpose." As the president of the American Academy of Forensic Sciences and president of the American College of Legal Medicine in 1971, I felt that I qualified.

For more than a year, I had written to the National Archives and Burke Marshall, the executor of the Kennedy archive materials, seeking to review the materials. My letters and phone calls went unanswered. The big breakthrough occurred in November 1971 when *New York Times* investigative reporter Fred Graham called me, saying he heard I had applied to be the first nongovernmental expert to review the official assassination materials.

I confirmed that I had, but I told him I was being stonewalled. Mr. Graham told me he would make a few calls to see if he could find out why. That is when I first came to fully recognize the power of the *New York Times*. Within days of Mr. Graham's call, Mr. Marshall called me back for the first time, and the wheels for me to examine the evidence were finally set in motion.

For two days I had exclusive access to all the physical evidence, autopsy materials, and crime scene photographs. I entered the National Archives a little skeptical of the official investigations into the assassination of President Kennedy. What I saw during those two days convinced me that the truth still remains unknown. Those two days changed my view about the honesty of my government.

As I studied the detailed inventory, my mind reflected back on November 22, 1963. At age thirty-two, I was the director of laboratory sciences and pathology at Leech Farm Veterans Hospital in Pittsburgh. At the same time, I was a junior partner at a law firm. I also had just accepted a position as Allegheny County assistant district attorney, advising prosecutors in homicide cases and working with the crime laboratory.

But on that particular day, I had traveled to Los Angeles for a medicolegal conference and decided to drop by the Los Angeles County coroner's office to see a new friend and colleague, Dr. Thomas Noguchi. At the time, Tom was the deputy coroner, though he would later be promoted to coroner and become well known for autopsies on Marilyn Monroe, John Belushi, Natalie Wood, and Robert Kennedy.

Tom and I were standing in one of his autopsy examination rooms, discussing where we should go for lunch, when his secretary walked in and whispered something in his ear.

"The president has been shot," Tom immediately stated. "He and the governor of Texas were shot in their motorcade in downtown Dallas. She [his secretary] doesn't know how bad it is. They've been rushed to the hospital."

Tom knew a restaurant down the street that had a television we could watch as we ate. It was the slowest meal I have ever eaten. For two emotional hours, we sat and watched CBS News anchor Walter Cronkite and then cub reporter Dan Rather explain what had happened and then interview witnesses and officials.

President and Mrs. Kennedy were visiting Texas with Vice President Lyndon Johnson as part of their election campaign kickoff. They had been in Houston the night before. The morning of November 22, President Kennedy spoke to the Fort Worth Chamber of Commerce. The president and first lady arrived at Love Field at 11:40 AM for a much-ballyhooed motorcade tour of downtown Dallas. Despite a weather forecast of rain, tens of thousands of Dallas citizens lined the streets.[1]

At 11:50 AM, the presidential motorcade, consisting of sixteen cars and a dozen motorcycles, exited the tarmac at Love Field for a ten-mile drive through the downtown area. The motorcade was led by a Dallas police squad car that traveled about a quarter mile ahead of the rest of the convoy, in an attempt to identify signs of trouble. Six Dallas police officers on motorcycles and an unmarked Dallas police car followed it.[2]

Approximately five car lengths behind was the presidential limo, a specially designed 1961 Lincoln Continental convertible. Mrs. Kennedy carried roses she had been given upon stepping off Air Force One in Dallas. She was seated next to President Kennedy in the backseat of the presidential limousine. Texas governor John Connally and his wife, Nellie, were seated in jump seats directly in front of the president and Mrs. Kennedy. Two Secret Service agents were in the front seat. Four Dallas police officers on motorcycles flanked the presidential limo.[3]

Directly behind the presidential limo was a car packed with eight Secret Service agents. Following that car was another limousine carrying Vice President Johnson and his wife, as well as Senator Ralph Yarborough of Texas. A series of cars followed, carrying more Secret Service agents, presidential staff, Adm. George Burkley (the president's personal physician), and journalists.

At President Kennedy's request, the Secret Service had removed the "bubble top" from the presidential limo. He wanted to be able to see the people of Texas, and he wanted them to see him. The Secret Service had been instructed by the president's political advisors to drive extremely slowly so people could get a good look at the president.

The motorcade slowed to about eleven miles per hour as it wound its way through downtown Dallas toward the Dallas Trade Mart, where the president was scheduled to give a speech. President and Mrs. Kennedy smiled and waved as the crowds on the sidewalks cheered and applauded. The president had twice ordered the Secret Service to stop the car to let him shake hands with schoolchildren lining the street.

The cars traveled down Main Street amid the tall buildings. The motorcade turned right onto Houston Street and then left onto Elm Street, taking it through the heart of Dealey Plaza. As the cars moved toward the Texas School Book Depository Building at 411 Elm Street, Mrs. Connally turned to comment on the incredible welcome, in response to the estimated quarter of a million people amassed to see the president that day.

"Mr. President, you can't say that Dallas doesn't love you," she stated.

"That is very obvious," responded President Kennedy, the final words he would ever speak.[4]

Only a few seconds later, at exactly 12:30 PM, shots were fired. President Kennedy's hand went to his neck. More shots sounded. A bullet struck the president in the head, spraying Mrs. Kennedy with blood.

"My God," she screamed out. "I've got his brains in my hands."[5]

"Oh my God," yelled Governor Connally, who had also been hit. "They're going to kill us all."[6]

Immediately, the motorcade sped away toward nearby Parkland Hospital, where emergency room doctors were alerted that the president and the governor had been injured and were on the way. The motorcade arrived at the hospital's rear entrance within five minutes. President Kennedy lay over in the back seat, his head in his wife's lap. Secret Service agents raced inside the emergency room to get stretchers. With the help of hospital technicians and nurses, they carried the governor and the president into emergency trauma rooms one and two. The president appeared to have at least two gunshot wounds—one to the back of the head and one to the front of the neck. Governor Connally appeared to have at least three gunshot wounds—one in the back that pierced through the right side of his chest, a second wound to his right wrist, and a third wound to his left thigh.

Doctors frantically worked to save President Kennedy's life. But there was no pulse, no blood pressure, and only a faint heartbeat. Their efforts were all in vain. Tom and I were watching the news when it was officially announced that President Kennedy had been declared dead at 1 PM Dallas time. Thirty-eight minutes later, President Kennedy's casket was loaded onto Air Force One and Lyndon Johnson was given the oath of office.

Tom and I were preparing to head back to his office about thirty minutes later when another news bulletin flashed on the screen. Walter Cronkite reported that Dallas police had arrested a man who they believed was responsible for the president's shooting. His name was Lee Harvey Oswald, a twenty-four-year-old man who worked in the Texas School Book Depository Building. Police said Oswald, an ex–US Marine, had also shot a Dallas police officer named J. D. Tippit in his attempt to escape. Police had tracked Oswald to the Texas Theatre, where he was arrested.

"I didn't shoot nobody," Oswald yelled to reporters as he was paraded before the television and newspaper cameras.

Speaking to reporters late that afternoon, Dallas County district attorney Henry Wade fueled speculation of a conspiracy when he said he suspected there was more than one shooter. Initial news reports indicated that there may have been two shooters—one firing at the president from behind, possibly from an open window in the School Book Depository, and a second person shooting from an area in front of the car.

In the early morning hours of November 23, authorities officially charged Oswald with the murder of President Kennedy. Federal law enforcement officials stated that they had identified the Italian-manufactured 2766 Mannlicher-Carcano rifle used to shoot the president as belonging to Oswald. The authorities also publicly announced that Oswald was a Communist sympathizer and a crazed man who acted alone in killing the president.

Even so, Oswald proclaimed his innocence and demanded to see a lawyer. But he would never get the opportunity to tell his story or dispute the evidence against him. One day later, on November 24, Oswald was shot and killed on live network television as he was being transferred from the Dallas City Jail to the Dallas County Jail. Dallas nightclub owner Jack Ruby, who reportedly had ties to organized crime, had somehow slipped through security and shot Oswald at point-blank range. Photographers for the city's two newspapers, the *Dallas Morning News* and the *Dallas Times-Herald*, captured Ruby in the act of shooting. The *Times-Herald* photographer later won a Pulitzer Prize for his photograph.

There were those who were suspicious of the lone-gunman theory from day one. Rumors surfaced that the Mafia had ordered the shooting. Others thought that the Cubans or Communists were behind it. And there were even those who contended that the Central Intelligence Agency or Vice President Johnson were involved.

Under pressure to conduct a full, thorough, and independent investigation, President Johnson on November 29 signed Executive Order 11130, which created a special blue-ribbon commission to determine what exactly had happened a week earlier in Dallas. United States chief justice Earl Warren, whose integrity was beyond reproach, was appointed to lead the seven-member panel.

This body was given unprecedented investigative authority, including subpoena power and the ability to grant immunity from prosecution in return for testimony. The FBI, the Secret Service, and the CIA were ordered to cooperate with all the commission's information requests.

The panel's official title was the President's Commission on the Assassination of President John F. Kennedy, though it quickly developed a shorter name that would stick throughout the years: the Warren Commission. It interviewed 552 witnesses and reviewed more than twenty-five thousand pages of investigative reports from the FBI, the Secret Service, and the CIA.

In the end, the commission's ten-month investigation and subsequent findings relied heavily on three sources: a spectator's film that captured the entire incident, the original autopsy findings, and the investigative resources of the Federal Bureau of Investigation. The commission issued its twenty-six-volume, 888-page report on September 24, 1964. The Warren Commission concluded:

(1) Oswald was the lone assassin;
(2) three bullets were fired, all from the sixth floor of the Texas School Book Depository Building;
(3) the first bullet missed completely;
(4) the second bullet entered President Kennedy's upper back, exited his neck, then struck Governor Connally in the back, went through the right side of his chest, through his right wrist and finally into the governor's left thigh; and
(5) the third and fatal bullet struck President Kennedy in the head.

There was no conspiracy, no second shooter, no involvement by any government agency—US or foreign—according to the panel. Nor was organized crime involved. Just one crazed man. Oswald had been in the US Marine Corps when he became sympathetic to Communism and Cuba. In 1959 he traveled to Russia where he sought to defect. The Soviet Union granted Oswald's request, providing him a job and an apartment in Minsk, although not granting him citizenship. Three years later, Oswald apparently had a change of heart when he returned to the United States to live, bringing with him his new wife, Marina, whose uncle was a colonel in the KGB.

The Warren Commission's findings seemed reasonable to me. The only information I had about President Kennedy's assassination is what I gleaned from the newspapers and from television. I read about those who argued that there was a cover-up or a conspiracy, but I gave their claims little credence. My opinion was that conspiracy buffs were probably just supporters of President Kennedy who simply didn't want to accept the fact that their leader was dead or that he had been killed by a lone gunman.

After all, if there was evidence of a conspiracy, I figured Robert Kennedy, the president's brother and the attorney general of the United States, would have blown the whistle. If there had been a conspiracy to kill the president, surely the FBI or Congress would have made it public. Surely the news media—the *New York Times*, the *Washington Post*, or CBS News—would have discovered and unveiled any legitimate evidence of a conspiracy.

The following year I was asked by the program chairman of the American Academy of Forensic Sciences (AAFS) to present a critical review of the Warren Commission Report at the organization's annual meeting to be held in Chicago in February 1965. The AAFS is the principal national organization for professionals in various forensic scientific fields. The only way for me to obtain a copy of the Warren Commission report was at the Carnegie Library of Pittsburgh. No one was permitted to check out copies, so I spent every evening for two weeks reading key portions of the twenty-six-volume report.

As I stated earlier, the Warren Commission's findings were based largely on three sources: a homemade film, FBI investigative reports, and the autopsy.

The Warren Commission had reviewed more than five hundred still photographs and moving films that were taken in Dealey Plaza at about the time the president was assassinated. But the single most important piece of physical evidence, as cited by the panel, was a film taken by Dallas businessman Abraham Zapruder, a Russian-born immigrant who had captured the entire incident on tape. The report repeatedly pointed to the eight-millimeter film as decisive evidence in determining the number of shots fired, the sequence of the injuries to President Kennedy and Governor Connally, the trajectory of the bullets, and the number of gunmen. The film is about twenty-six seconds long and consists of 486 individual frames. The camera processed about 18.3 frames per second, meaning that the film caught the reactions of the president and governor every one-eighteenth of a second.

The film conclusively revealed, the Warren Commission reported, that President Kennedy and Governor Connally were struck by the same bullet, which was fired from behind, specifically from the Texas School Book Depository. "Although it is not necessary to any essential findings of the Commission to determine just which shot hit Governor Connally, there is persuasive evidence from the experts to indicate that the same bullet which pierced the President's throat also caused Governor Connally's wounds," the panel stated.[7]

The report asserted that the Zapruder film demonstrated that the second bullet that struck the president also came from the book depository building.

In 1965 I had no reason to question the commission's interpretation of the film. I believed the panel's conclusions for two reasons: the fact that the commission reported that the Zapruder film proved its findings that Oswald acted alone and the fact that the conclusions were unanimously agreed to by Chief Justice Warren, the six other respected commission members, and the FBI.

Besides, the physical evidence that connected Oswald to the shooting seemed quite overwhelming. I read that the FBI had documented that Oswald had purchased the Mannlicher-Carcano by mail order a few weeks before the shooting. The FBI discovered a photograph that featured Oswald holding the murder weapon. And authorities recovered three empty bullet shells in the so-called sniper's nest, near the sixth-floor window in the school depository building. Pretty damning evidence, or so it seemed at the time.

My intent was not to question the findings of the Warren Commission, but to review how the autopsy and other medicolegal aspects of the inquiry were conducted. In doing so, I became simply astonished.

The first problem occurred just minutes after doctors at Parkland Hospital declared President Kennedy dead. The Secret Service announced that they were removing the body from the hospital and taking it to Air Force One, where it would be flown to Washington, DC, for examination. As the agents were in the process of taking the president's corpse from the hospital, they were confronted by the Dallas County medical examiner, Dr. Earl Rose. A forensic pathologist who was well respected in the medicolegal community, Dr. Rose ordered the Secret Service to stop.

A homicide had occurred in Dallas County. At the time, there were no federal laws that criminalized murder. Instead, homicide was exclusively a state law issue. As such, Texas law provided that the bodies of homicide victims fell under the exclusive control of the duly elected county coroner. In this case, that was Dr. Rose.

However, Secret Service agents ignored Dr. Rose's pleas. They forced the medical examiner aside and pushed the president's body toward a waiting ambulance. Dr. Rose could have gone to state or federal court to halt the removal of the body. But everything was moving so fast, he probably realized that there wasn't time to file the emergency petition and conduct a hearing. In actuality, even if Dr. Rose and Dallas law enforcement had obtained a court order, I'm not sure that President Johnson would have agreed to abide by it.[8]

So what? You may ask.

What difference does it make that the body was flown out of Texas to Washington, DC, for examination?

At this point, Lee Harvey Oswald was still alive. He was just being arrested and transported to the city jail for questioning. If Oswald had not been murdered by Jack Ruby, Oswald would have been put on trial for the crime of murder. Such a trial would have taken place in Dallas because the Sixth Amendment of the US Constitution requires that people be tried in the jurisdiction where the crime takes place. In addition, the law requires that state authorities retain control of the evidence to guarantee its authenticity. By removing the body from the supervision and control of the Dallas County coroner, federal officials probably destroyed the admissibility of any evidence gained through the autopsy. In a gunshot death, the autopsy is extremely important in determining how many bullets struck the body, where the bullets came from, the trajectory of the bullets, and proof that the bullet wounds were indeed the cause of death.

Air Force One landed at Andrews Air Force Base just before 6 PM eastern time, according to the Warren Commission report. The president's body was then transported to Bethesda Hospital. Dr. James Humes, the thirty-nine-year-old director of the Bethesda Naval Medical School's laboratory services; Dr. J. Thornton Boswell, the hospital's chief of pathology; and Dr. Pierre Finck, an army colonel and pathologist who had an expertise in ballistics, were chosen to perform the most important autopsy in our nation's history.

All three were military officers. All three were fine men and probably good doctors and good soldiers. However, Humes and Boswell were not forensic pathologists. Neither of them had ever performed an autopsy involving gunshot wounds. Finck was a forensic pathologist, but he had not functioned in the position of a forensic pathologist in any coroner's office. Not a single person in the autopsy room had the education, or the training, or the experience to handle the task that faced them.

Why is the issue of a forensic pathologist performing the autopsy so important? We have to look no further than the initial component of the autopsy, referred to as the external examination. Drs. Humes and Boswell started prior to Dr. Finck's arrival, which should not have happened. When they did commence the autopsy, they totally missed the fact that President Kennedy had a bullet wound in the front of his neck. They completely failed to mention it when they gave their oral autopsy findings to the FBI that evening.

The reason that they missed the bullet wound in the front of the neck was simple: the three Bethesda pathologists did not contact the doctors at Parkland Hospital who worked on the president in their efforts to save his life. "Forensic pathology 101" makes it clear that the pathologist should speak to the emergency room physicians prior to conducting an autopsy on a victim of bullet or stab wounds. If Drs. Humes, Boswell, and Finck had talked with the emergency room physicians, they would have discovered that President Kennedy had a bullet wound in his neck. However, the emergency room doctors had to enlarge the wound by performing a tracheotomy in an effort to get oxygen to the president's lungs. When the emergency room doctors did the tracheotomy, they destroyed nearly all of the original markings of the gunshot wound. This is not to criticize the Parkland doctors in pointing this out. They did all they could to save the president's life.

By the pathologists not knowing there was a gunshot wound to the neck, however, they did not trace the path of the bullet or examine the neck area to see if the wound was caused by a bullet entering or exiting the body. The pathologists did not find out about the neck wound until the next day. That is unacceptable and inexcusable.

Similarly, I was shocked and appalled to learn that the pathologists did not dissect and trace the bullet wound in President Kennedy's back. Because the pathologists were unaware of the neck wound, they concluded that the bullet must have been forced out of the entrance wound in the president's back when the emergency room doctors had applied pressure to the front of his chest in their resuscitation efforts. Who gave the order not to track the path of the bullet through the body and why? I've never heard a legitimate or official explanation from anyone who knows the answer.

Because the brain is comprised of soft tissue, it could not be properly examined right away. The pathologists placed it in formalin, a fixative solution that allows the brain matter to harden. The formalin causes the brain to go from being like a soft-boiled egg to having the consistency of a hard-boiled egg. However, the pathologists did not perform an adequate examination of the brain when they looked at it two weeks later. The pathologists should have serially sectioned the brain, which would have allowed them to track the path of the bullet that struck the president in the head.

The bullet to the head was what the pathologists concluded had killed him. Yet they did not dissect the brain. I was flabbergasted. There was simply no excuse for this. I am as appalled today as when I first learned this information four decades ago.

But there's more that is equally disturbing. Dr. Humes announced a few months later that he had burned his original autopsy notes in his home fireplace two days after the autopsy.[9] Prosecutors, defense lawyers, and judges make it clear that pathologists in criminal investigations should keep copies of their original autopsy notes. It is part of the legal discovery process in a criminal or civil case. Why did he destroy them? Were there discrepancies or mistakes that might have been revealed in his notes?

I became equally as critical of the police investigation of the case. First, the crime scene was very poorly contained. Witnesses were allowed to leave the scene without being questioned or identified. The president's limousine was not properly quarantined and examined for forensic evidence. Amazingly, Governor Connally's clothes were laundered before they could be examined by investigators. If the bullet that entered President Kennedy's back and exited his neck had also struck Governor Connally, as the Warren Commission claimed, having the governor's clothes would have helped prove it, because it is likely that some of the president's blood or bodily tissue would have been deposited on the governor's clothes.

Nonetheless, I concluded my presentation without questioning the basic findings of the Warren Commission in any way. Critiquing the conclusions of the Warren Commission was not my charge. Even if it had been, I'm not sure I would have done so, because I didn't have sufficient evidence or reason to believe the commission was wrong in deciding that Oswald was the lone gunman.

I was quite critical, however, regarding the autopsy and the forensic investigation. In fact, I stated that if Oswald had survived and if the state would have had to put him on trial for the murder of President Kennedy, prosecutors would have lost the case. The medical and forensic evidence was so screwed up, so incomplete, and so tainted that it would not have held up as legitimate in a court of law.

Following my lecture, a moment presented itself that I will never forget. Dr. Pierre Finck, one of the pathologists who had performed the autopsy, approached me during a breakfast meeting to congratulate me on my paper. Dr. Finck could have told me I was off base with my conclusions. Dr. Finck could have told me that I had it all wrong. Dr. Finck could have defended the autopsy of President Kennedy as proper and adequate. But he didn't. I will never forget his comments. "You cannot believe what it was like," he told me that wintry morning in Chicago. "It was horrible. Horrible. I only wish I could tell you about it."

Later, in 1972, as I sat in the National Archives Building reviewing the physical and medical evidence, I regretted that I had not pushed Dr. Finck a little more to give me some details. But I didn't. In 1965, as I shook Dr. Finck's hand, I believed that I had said all I would ever say publicly about the investigation into the assassination of President Kennedy.

How wrong I was.

As I scanned down the list of items connected to the Kennedy assassination that were stored at the National Archives, I noticed an original copy of the Zapruder film. Mr. Johnson, the archivist, told me that he had a projector set up for me to review the film if I wished. He added that the film was only about thirty seconds long. He said that while more than five hundred photographs and pieces of film recorded portions of the assassination, only the Zapruder film captured the entire event on tape. When he informed me that the film was graphic, I reminded him that I'm a forensic pathologist and used to witnessing the results of violence and tragedy.

What I didn't tell Mr. Johnson was that I had seen the Zapruder film before. In 1966 I received a call from Dr. Josiah Thompson, a Haverford University professor who was working on an article on the Kennedy assassination for *Life* magazine. Dr. Thompson told me that the editors at *Life* had purchased an original copy of the Zapruder film and that they wanted me to fly to New York to watch the eight-millimeter film with them. The film had never been shown publicly, though *Life* had published several still photographs in its magazine. Of course, I had read about the film in the newspaper, seen the few photographs that *Life* had chosen to publish, and studied additional photographs from the film published in the Warren Commission report. I was acutely aware how important the film was in determining what had happened in Dealey Plaza.

I agreed to assist, and a few days later I flew to New York and met with Dr. Thompson and the editors of *Life* magazine. We watched the film, which was twenty-six seconds long. Dr. Thompson explained to me that the film was taken with a Bell & Howell Model 414PD Zoomatic Director Series camera. The film was 8 mm Kodachrome color but recorded no sound. It consisted of 486 frames, which played at a speed of 18.3 frames per second. Mr. Zapruder, who operated a clothing manufacturing business in Dallas, wasn't even sure he had captured the shooting on tape. As the motorcade approached from Houston Street, Zapruder climbed onto a concrete abutment about seventy feet from the middle of Elm Street, where the president's limousine would pass.

A reporter for the *Dallas Morning News*, realizing the potential importance of the film, contacted Secret Service agents, who escorted Zapruder immediately to a Kodak film store, where they watched it for the first time. Zapruder had the store make three copies. He kept the original, gave two copies to Secret Service agents on November 22, and sold a copy to *Life* for $150,000—a tidy sum of cash in those days.

The importance of the Zapruder film is that it shows President Kennedy and Governor Connally as they were being shot. To better examine the timing and sequence of the event, *Life* magazine printed each frame into eleven-by-fifteen-inch photographs. It allowed readers to inspect each movement, each expression, and each reaction at one-eighteenth-second intervals.

On Thursday, August 24, 1972, I sat alone in the National Archives watching the film and examining the still enlargements of each frame. The first part of the film shows Zapruder, called "Mr. Z" by his staff, taping his employees as they waited on the grassy knoll for the presidential motorcade. Zapruder then turned off his camera until the president's limo was in sight.

The film begins at frame 140, as the car carrying President and Mrs. Kennedy, as well as Governor and Mrs. Connally, turns onto Elm Street. Some JFK assassination researchers say the first shot, which reportedly missed, was fired between frames 151 and 153. The president, in frames 154 and 155, is shown turning his head from left to right.

The film shows, from frames 167 through 210, that foliage from the trees along Elm Street blocked the view that anyone would have had from the Texas School Book Depository Building. Frame 200 displays President Kennedy continuing to wave to onlookers, and no one in the car appears to have been shot.

Frame 210 is the first opportunity that a gunman from the

School Book Depository would have had to shoot at the president, who is shown leaning slightly forward. Frames 225 and 226 reveal President Kennedy moving his right arm from the side of the car and placing his hand to his throat. At this point, Governor Connally shows no sign of being struck.

In frame 230 Governor Connally is seen still tightly grasping his large white Stetson hat with his right hand. His face reveals no signs of pain or of being hit. Yet the bullet that struck Connally shattered his right wrist and severed his radius bone. The Texas governor's first visible reaction to being shot comes in frames 235 and 236, when his mouth opens wide. After viewing the Zapruder film, Connally told the Warren Commission that he believed he had been shot between frames 231 and 234.

As I studied the photographs, I remembered that the government's tests of the Mannlicher-Carcano rifle that Oswald allegedly used showed that it would have taken him a minimum of 2.3 seconds to fire a bullet, reload, and fire again. And this did not even factor in his reaiming the rifle. Taking into account that the bullets from the Mannlicher-Carcano rifle traveled at a speed exceeding two thousand feet per second, I started having serious doubts in 1966 about the so-called single-bullet theory after watching the Zapruder film for the first time.

The single-bullet theory holds that the missile entered President Kennedy's back, coursed through the front of his neck, entered Governor Connally's back, exited from the front of his chest, reentered the governor's right wrist, exited from the front of his wrist, and then reentered his left thigh. The bullet, according to the final Warren Commission report, apparently fell out of the governor's left thigh while he was on a stretcher at Parkland Hospital. The bullet was found quite fortuitously an hour and a half later by a maintenance person at Parkland Hospital who was trying to get to the bathroom. When he bent down to move the stretchers in the ER corridor, he discovered a bullet that no one else had seen.

If the same bullet that struck President Kennedy also struck Governor Connally, then the governor's reaction should have been considerably earlier, nearly simultaneous with the reactions of President Kennedy. Yet the Warren Commission was contending that approximately a second and a half after being shot in the upper right back, after having a rib fractured, after having his wrist bone shattered, and after having the bullet enter his left thigh, Governor Connally showed no sign of being injured.

Highly unlikely. With those kinds of injuries, the governor would have exhibited an immediate response.

Frames 312 and 313 show the right side area (known as the occipital area) of President Kennedy's head exploding, creating a pink cloud of blood around his head and scattering chunks of brain and bone. Then his head lurches backward and to the left. His body stiffens. The following three frames show a Dallas police officer riding on a motorcycle behind the president's limousine being sprayed with blood and brain matter.

As I watched the film over and over and reviewed the still photographs, I realized a couple of different things regarding the Warren Commission report: the panel was correct in declaring that the Zapruder film is the best documentary evidence of the Kennedy assassination; however, the film contradicted some conclusions of the Warren Commission.

First, the film calls into question the timing of the bullet that reportedly struck President Kennedy and Governor Connally. If the president was struck in frame 210, as the Warren Commission contended, then more than a second elapsed before Governor Connally was struck. That is not consistent with a bullet traveling at a speed of two thousand feet per second.

Second, firearms experts said it would take 2.3 seconds for Oswald to have fired the Mannlicher-Carcano, reloaded, and fired again—far too little time for Oswald to have shot the president and the governor with the same gun.

Third, the film also casts doubt on the trajectory of the bullet.

The single-bullet theory, as proposed by the Warren Commission, holds that one missile, known as Commission Exhibit 399, entered the president's back, coursed through the upper portion of his back and neck without striking any bone or cartilage, and then exited from the front of the neck in the midline near the level of the knot of a tie. The same bullet reentered Governor Connally's back and broke the right fifth rib, destroying four inches of that bone. The bullet exited from the front of Governor Connally's chest below the right nipple. The same bullet reentered the back of Governor Connally's wrist, causing a comminuted or fragmented fracture of the distal end of the radius, which is one of the two large bones that comes down from the elbow to the wrist. The bullet finally exited from the front of Governor Connally's right wrist and re-entered Governor Connally's left thigh.

But as I viewed the Zapruder film and looked at the still photographs, I realized something was wrong. A bullet fired from the sixth-floor window of the Texas School Book Depository Building toward President Kennedy in frame 210 would have been traveling at a downward angle of about seventeen degrees, from back to front, and from right to left, as it entered his back. A bullet travels in a straight line, unless it strikes an object that causes the projectile to alter course.

With that in mind, if the bullet was shot by Oswald from the sixth floor, it would have been traveling at a downward trajectory and from right to left. If the bullet didn't hit any bones in the president's back, chest, or neck, the president needed to be dramatically leaning forward with his head almost on his knees for the bullet to have exited through his neck. The Zapruder film clearly shows President Kennedy sitting nearly bolt upright.

But I digress with facts and logic.

If you draw a straight line from President Kennedy's back at the point of entrance and the front of the neck at the level of the knot of a tie, as shown in the Zapruder film, the bullet would probably miss Governor Connally completely or possibly have clipped him in the left back or left shoulder area, instead of the right armpit. The film shows the governor sitting directly in front of the president.

For this bullet to have done what the Warren Commission contended, the bullet would have had to emerge from the president's neck, stop in midair, make an acute turn to the right about eighteen to twenty inches, stop again in midair, and turn downward and enter the governor's back on the right side, just behind the right armpit. The angle downward through Governor Connally's chest is about twenty-two degrees, while the angle from the wrist and into the thigh is about forty-five degrees.

Four years of college, four years of medical school, six years of additional education and training to become a forensic pathologist, three years of law school, and nearly a decade of experience has led me to understand one basic principle: bullets travel in straight lines. Bullets do not change course in midair. As I considered the horizontal and vertical gyrations that this wondrous missile must have accomplished, I began to label it the "magic bullet."

It was then that I suddenly realized how special this bullet really was. This is the slug that was found on a stretcher by a maintenance man at Parkland Hospital hours after President Kennedy and Governor Connally had been first wheeled in. How did the Warren Commission develop this theory? Initially, federal authorities didn't know about the president's wound in the neck. So they contended that the bullet must have come from President Kennedy's back as the Parkland doctors were trying to save his life. When the autopsy doctors and investigators learned the next day about the bullet wound to the president's neck, they decided that the bullet must have entered his back and exited his neck. Under their original theory, this bullet, which traveled at a speed of two thousand feet per second, did not have the power to penetrate the starched collar. That is some heavy starch.

Then along came the Warren Commission with a second scenario. In order to make the facts fit the theory that Oswald was the

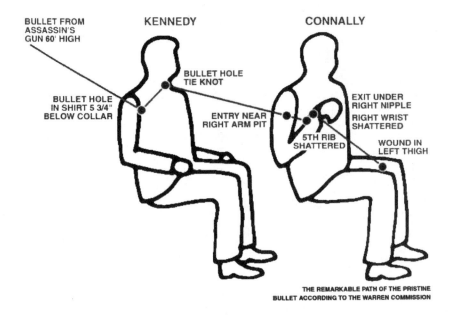

BULLET FROM ASSASSIN'S GUN 60' HIGH

KENNEDY

CONNALLY

BULLET HOLE TIE KNOT

BULLET HOLE IN SHIRT 5 3/4" BELOW COLLAR

ENTRY NEAR RIGHT ARM PIT

EXIT UNDER RIGHT NIPPLE

RIGHT WRIST SHATTERED

5TH RIB SHATTERED

WOUND IN LEFT THIGH

THE REMARKABLE PATH OF THE PRISTINE BULLET ACCORDING TO THE WARREN COMMISSION

lone gunman, the panel needed to develop a scenario in which only three bullets were fired from the sixth-floor window of the book depository building, and the shots had to take place during the time period framed by the Zapruder film. Arlen Specter, a young but brilliant lawyer serving as one of the junior counsel members of the Warren Commission, came up with a scenario that fit. But it required that all the nonfatal wounds from President Kennedy and Governor Connally were caused by the same bullet.

And then there's the business of the bullet just popping out of Governor Connally's left thigh while he was lying on the stretcher at Parkland Hospital. This is a substantial piece of metal that was buried deep in the governor's thigh near the femur. The entrance hole in the skin was small. There is no way that a bullet that went down that deep would just come back out. A bullet will on rare occasions plop out of an entrance wound if the hole is a large gaping wound with extensively torn tissues. But in wounds such as the one suffered by Governor Connally in the left thigh, bullets become immediately entrapped in hemorrhagic tissue. The tissue swells and the skin, which stretches to accommodate the entry of the bullet, becomes elastic-like within a few seconds, entrapping the bullet in the tissue.

At this point, I asked Mr. Johnson if I could examine CE 399, the "magic bullet." A few minutes later, he brought it to me in a small case. The bullet was resting on a bed of cotton padding. I picked up the bullet and held it against the light. It was in nearly pristine condition. The bullet, before it was shot, weighed 161 grains. But the bullet I held in my fingers weighed 158.6 grains.

I immediately recognized that that was impossible. It was impossible for a bullet to do what the Warren Commission claimed that this bullet did—striking President Kennedy in the back, exiting his neck, breaking Governor Connally's fifth right rib, shattering the radius bone in his wrist, and entering his left thigh—and lose only 1.5 percent of its weight and not be more deformed. Bullet fragments could be seen in the x-rays taken of Governor Connally's chest, wrist, and thighs.

Even the autopsy pathologists agreed with me on this point. Dr. Pierre Finck was asked by Arlen Specter during the Warren Commission hearings if CE 399 "could have been the bullet which inflicted the wound on Governor Connally's right wrist?"

"No, for the reason that there are too many fragments described in that wrist," Dr. Finck responded. "There was practically no loss of this bullet."[10]

In fact, the federal government did an experiment trying to re-create the magic bullet at the US Army's Edgewood Arsenal in Maryland.[11] They shot Mannlicher-Carcano bullets through goat carcasses and human cadavers, breaking one rib in the goat's chest and finally breaking the distal end of the radius in the human cadavers to simulate the fractures in Connally. They also fired identical bullets into cotton wadding only. The bullets that broke the rib of the goat showed significant deformity. The bullets that broke the radius of different cadavers show tremendous deformity. Some of the bullets fragmented and all demonstrated the mushrooming, umbrella-like appearance seen in bullets that impact dense bones. Keep in mind that none of those bullets in the experiment broke both bones, as the alleged magic bullet did. The Warren Commission's own experiment proved the single-bullet theory to be physically impossible.

As I looked at CE 399, I realized one thing: this was indeed a magic bullet—magic because it accommodated the Warren Commission's every wish and desire. There has never been a bullet like this one in the world.

Among the many documents I came upon was a verbatim transcript of a press briefing that the emergency room doctors at Parkland Hospital conducted at 3:16 PM, just two hours after the president had been pronounced dead. Dr. Malcolm Perry and neurosurgeon Dr. Kemp Clark discussed what they had witnessed.

Reporter: Where was the entrance wound?

Dr. Perry: There was an entrance wound in the neck.

Reporter: Which way was the bullet coming on the neck wound?

Dr. Perry: It appeared to be coming at him.

Reporter: Doctor, describe the entrance wound.

Dr. Perry: The wound appeared to be an entrance wound in the front of the throat.[12]

As I scanned through some of the five hundred or more photographs taken that day at Dealey Plaza, I happened to examine those taken of the Texas School Book Depository Building. There were some photographs that showed the presidential motorcade turning from Main Street onto Houston Street, heading directly toward the School Book Depository. I couldn't help but think that if Oswald was the lone gunman, why didn't he shoot when the president's limo was on Houston Street directly in front of him? The view from the sixth floor of the School Book Depository Building of the motorcade coming directly down Houston Street was unobstructed by trees or foliage. It was a much clearer shot. Instead, the commission claimed that Oswald waited until the limo was partially hidden by tree branches and leaves and at a more difficult angle to hit a moving target. It doesn't make sense.

Over the next several hours, I examined the Mannlicher-Carcano rifle and the three spent bullet shell casings. I'm not a gun expert, but I can tell you that this was not a very sophisticated weapon. It's weighty and bulky, and it is not easy to fire and reload. It is considered by gun experts to be the most inferior weapon of its genre in existence at that time.

I also examined the president's clothes. His shirt, pants, and jacket were neatly folded and separated from each other by thin soft paper. I held up his suit jacket to examine the bullet hole. It was approximately five and three-quarter inches down from the base of the back. This raised another interesting issue. Where was the entrance wound in President Kennedy's back?

The autopsy doctors initially placed the bullet entry wound farther down on the president's back, about five and three-quarter inches from the base of the neck. The two Secret Service agents who had the first contact with President Kennedy immediately after the shooting, Glenn Bennett and Clint Hill, told the Warren Commission that the bullet wound was four to six inches below the neckline on the right side of the spinal column, which is exactly where the original autopsy notes indicate it was.[13] Even the FBI agents who witnessed the autopsy reported that the back wound was "below the shoulders." The agents, in their report which was sealed until a few years ago, stated that they doubted that the same bullet that entered the back could have been the bullet that exited the neck, because the entrance wound was too low on the back.[14]

In order to support the single-bullet theory, Warren Commission loyalists claim that the bullet wound on the president's back was actually four inches higher. That would make the theory that the same bullet which entered President Kennedy's back also exited his neck more feasible, though still highly unlikely. They also keep moving Governor Connally farther and farther to the left, even though the Zapruder film and eyewitnesses confirm that he was seated directly in front of the president. If they edge the governor over any farther in their hypothesis, they will have him sitting in Mrs. Connally's lap.

My attention returned for a few minutes to frames 312 and 313 of the Zapruder film. They show President Kennedy sitting in a slight chin-downward position as the fatal bullet strikes his head. The frames show blood and brain matter being sprayed on Mrs. Kennedy, on the back of the presidential limousine, and on the Dallas police officers who followed their car.

If the bullet was fired from behind, why did the president's head lurch backward at the point of the bullet's impact, instead of forward with the direction and momentum of the bullet? Also, why is nearly all the blood and brain matter being sprayed toward the back of the car if the bullet was fired from behind the president? None of this seemed to make sense.

Indeed, the size and location of the fatal head wound, which were instrumental in determining the position of the gunman, were also in dispute. The truth is, very little about the evidence in this case is not in dispute.

The emergency room physicians at Parkland and the three autopsy pathologists agreed that the massive, fatal head wound was toward the back right side of the skull. The bullet, they said, entered at the base of the rear of the president's skull and exited on the right side of his head.

However, the size and location of the head wound officially changed in 1968. A panel appointed by then US attorney general Ramsey Clark reexamined the autopsy records and determined that President Kennedy's wound was actually four inches higher on his head than either the emergency room doctors or the autopsy pathologists had indicated. The Clark panel said it was a simple and easy mistake made by the original pathologists and that the higher head wound proved that the fatal shot was fired from the

Texas School Book Depository. The Clark panel based its findings exclusively on its review of the autopsy photographs and x-rays.

The problem, of course, is that the head wound described by the Clark panel was so significantly different from the wound described by the emergency room doctors and the autopsy pathologists. The emergency room doctors stated they saw cerebellar tissue when they examined the president's head. The cerebellum is located lower on the head, nowhere near the newly designated site of the entrance.

This modification or rediscovering of the official location of the wounds intrigued me.

"Are you ready for another item?" asked Mr. Johnson, who was at all times polite and extremely meticulous.

"Yes, I'm ready to review the autopsy materials," I replied. "Let's start with the original autopsy report and photographs, please."

The original autopsy describes the entrance point as "just above" the external occipital protuberance, which is the bony knob at the bottom rear of the skull.[15] While the autopsy pathologists did not say specifically how far above the external occipital protuberance, it is certain that they were not saying four inches. The exit wound was described as blowing out the back right side of the president's head, also known as the "parietal-temporal area."

While I may be critical of the three autopsy pathologists' lack of forensic pathology expertise, I do not believe they would have mistaken the back of President Kennedy's head for the top of his head.

But as I examined the autopsy photographs and x-rays, I discovered a couple of previously unreported items. The x-rays revealed a very dense 6.5-millimeter object positioned at the base of the skull. It was nine centimeters above the external occipital protuberance and one centimeter below a crack in the parietal bone in the skull. It was a large bullet fragment that was not mentioned in the autopsy report. Equally as baffling is why the autopsy pathologists did not retrieve this bullet fragment, as they did several much smaller fragments.

In addition, I spotted a small flap on the back of the president's head slightly above the neckline that appeared to be loose tissue. Was it an entrance wound or an exit wound that had not previously been reported?

If it was an entrance wound, it would prove the lone-gunman theory to be obsolete because it would require an additional bullet having been fired at President Kennedy. The Zapruder film confines the shooting to six seconds. And the Warren Commission's own testing, as I mentioned earlier, proves that Oswald could have fired only three bullets during the time allotted. If the flap is evidence of an exit wound, then it also disproves the lone-gunman theory, because it shows the bullet was fired from the front, probably entering the president's neck and exiting the back of his head.

Unfortunately, there is only one way to know for sure if this is an entrance or exit wound: to exhume the body of President Kennedy and conduct a second autopsy. I knew then and I know today that neither the Kennedy family nor the federal government will allow that to happen. At least not in my lifetime.

Something else seemed odd in the autopsy photographs of the head: there was very short but thick hair covering the spot on the president's head where the Parkland doctors claimed that there was a gaping hole from the bullet wound. The hair was less than an inch long in the photographs, even though this was a spot on the president's head where the hair would have been much longer. Instead, this was the length of hair that normally is found at the bottom of the scalp. It made me wonder if either President Kennedy's head or the autopsy photographs had been tampered with to cover up the actual wounds. Without examining the actual body, of course, I could not know for sure.

Among the autopsy photographs that Mr. Johnson brought to me was a roll of film that had been improperly exposed and ruined. I learned that an autopsy photographer who worked at Bethesda Naval Hospital took a series of pictures as the pathologists were starting their autopsy. However, a military official seized the camera, claiming the autopsy photographer was not authorized to take the pictures, and immediately stripped the film from the camera, which caused it to be overexposed. This roll of film reminded me of Dr. Finck's comments regarding how horrible the conditions were that night of the autopsy.

I also spent a considerable amount of time reviewing the x-rays taken by Parkland Hospital officials of Governor Connally's injuries. The x-rays showed bone injuries and fractures to the governor's right fifth rib and right radius above the wrist. Also clearly visible on the x-rays were small bullet fragments embedded in the governor's chest, right wrist, and left thigh. These bullet fragments were never removed. If they had been, tests could have been done to prove or disprove that they came from the so-called magic bullet. This was evidence of another gaffe by investigators.

As my time at the National Archives was running out, I had only three additional items I wished to review: the president's brain, autopsy photographs of the president's chest wounds, and microscopic tissue slides of the wounds.

The autopsy pathologists removed the brain from the skull during the autopsy the night of November 22, 1963. They placed the brain in a container of formalin for preservation for future dissection and examination. The brain is soft scrambled tissue, much like a soft-boiled egg. As noted earlier, the formalin causes the brain matter to harden, much like a hard-boiled egg. It usually takes about ten days to two weeks for this to occur. Once the brain tissue hardens, pathologists are able to dissect the brain to determine bullet trajectories. However, President Kennedy's brain had not been dissected. Nonetheless, I thought, at least it had been preserved for future examination.

The microscopic slides included sections of the actual wounds. I would have been able to tell from the skin tissue if the wounds were entrance or exit wounds. The sections on the slides would reveal the outer layer of the skin, which is called the epidermis. If the epidermis was pushed in, then it was an entrance wound. If it was an exit wound, the epidermis would be pushing out. There are also additional differentiating microscopic features between entrance and exit wounds.

But that is when Mr. Johnson told me the shocker: President Kennedy's brain, some x-rays of the chest, and the microscopic tissue slides were missing. Gone. Taken.

The Warren Commission report states that the brain was "removed and preserved for further study." The brain, the x-rays, and the microscopic slides were placed in a metal container for storage among the other Kennedy assassination materials presented to Mrs. Kennedy, though there is no evidence she ever received these materials. Instead, the assassination materials were stored for about a year by the president's personal secretary, Evelyn Lincoln, and his brother, Robert Kennedy. Mr. Johnson told me that when the Kennedy family decided to turn all the assassination materials over to the National Archives as a gift, the brain, chest x-rays, and microscopic slides were mysteriously not included. He told me he had no idea what happened to them, who had them, or when they disappeared.

Think about what is missing—the brain, the photos of the chest wound, and the slides. These are key pieces of hard physical evidence. Much of this case is subjective interpretation or circumstantial. But the evidence that is missing is actual physical evidence that cannot be duplicated.

Late that Friday afternoon, as I left the National Archives after spending two full days examining the evidence in the Kennedy assassination, I was met by Fred Graham of the *New York Times*. Mr. Graham had asked me to discuss my findings and observations with him, which I was happy to do since he was so instrumental in my gaining access to the materials. I told him about the missing brain and other materials, as well as my general opinion regarding the physical and medical evidence. That Sunday, August 27, the *New York Times* published a front-page article by Mr. Graham in which he detailed my findings.[16]

My interest and involvement in the assassination of President

Kennedy did not end with those two days at the National Archives. In 1975, amid growing public dissatisfaction with the outcome of the investigation in the murder of President Kennedy, President Gerald Ford, who had been an original member of the Warren Commission, created a new panel, headed by Vice President Nelson Rockefeller.

One of the panel's senior lawyers interviewed me regarding my scientific opinions. For five hours I walked the attorneys through my critique of the autopsy and my analysis of the medical and physical evidence. I testified that the evidence made it clear to me that the single-bullet theory was nonsense; that all the bullets were not fired from behind; that more than three shots were fired at President Kennedy and Governor Connally; that the autopsy was a sham; that I had become convinced there was a second gunman; and that the case should be reopened and reinvestigated.

Imagine my surprise when I read the Rockefeller Commission's report that I concurred with its opinion that all of the shots were indeed fired from behind and most likely from the Texas School Book Depository. The report stated that this was all the evidence that I had provided to the commission.

When I demanded to see a transcript of my testimony, I was told that it was considered confidential and that releasing my statement in full would be a breach of national security. I was stunned and dumbfounded. My statement was a matter of national security. I never thought that I was so important.

"If that transcript shows in any way that I have withdrawn or revised my thoughts of the Warren Commission Report, I'll eat the transcript on the steps of the White House," I told a reporter for the Associated Press.[17]

Twenty years later, the federal government finally released the transcript of my entire five-hour interview, and it showed exactly what I had stated.[18]

Two years later Congress created the House Select Committee on Assassinations, which was charged with reopening the investigations into the deaths of President Kennedy and Dr. Martin Luther King. To help acquire, organize, and analyze the medical and physical evidence in the Kennedy case, the committee appointed a nine-member pathology panel. I was surprised when I was asked to be one of the nine expert pathologists on the panel. In fact, I later learned from personal friends that considerable pressure had been applied to keep me from being appointed.

For several months we reviewed and discussed the evidence. Everyone agreed that the autopsy performed by the three military pathologists was woefully substandard. And all nine of us agreed that the forensic investigation was equally tragic.

However, I was alone in arguing that the single-bullet theory was scientifically absurd. I was alone in contending that there was more than one gunman. I was alone in believing that at least one, and possibly two, of the gunshots were fired from the front right side.

The other eight forensic pathologists were very qualified and very experienced. I simply believe they had made up their minds long ago that the Warren Commission was probably correct, and, as a result, their eyes were closed to accepting a different explanation.

During one of our panel discussions, I challenged my eight colleagues on the panel to show me another bullet that can match the condition and weight of the so-called magic bullet. "Go back to your respective cities and search through the thousands and thousands of bullets and show me one bullet that has done what you say this bullet has done and looks like this bullet looks," I implored the panel.

Twenty-seven years later, I'm still waiting.

My gut feeling was that the House Select Committee would whitewash its investigation, too. I was surprised when the committee's final report declared that there was a high degree of probability that President Kennedy's death was the result of a conspiracy that involved a second gunman. The committee report pointed to the Mafia as having the motive and means to organize the assassination plot.

The House Select Committee also stated that it was clear that senior government officials were determined that the outcome of any investigation should point to Oswald as the only gunman: "It must be said that the FBI generally exhausted its resources in confirming its case against Oswald as the lone assassin, a case that Director J. Edgar Hoover, at least, seemed determined to make within twenty-four hours of the assassination."[19]

As part of the committee's report, it turned over all its findings to the FBI and the US Department of Justice for further investigation. Unfortunately, the Justice Department was not interested or willing to continue the inquiry.

So what happened? Was there a conspiracy? How many gunmen were there? How many shots were fired?

There are truly two elements to consider. First, I do believe that there was a conspiracy to kill the president. I believe the physical, medical, and scientific evidence clearly points to at least two shooters. If there are two shooters, then there is, under the law, a "conspiracy." I also believe there were at least four shots fired, maybe five. Three bullets were probably fired from behind and probably two from the front.

I have never believed nor have I ever contended that the murder was the result of an official FBI or CIA planned assassination. However, I do believe that the assassination of President Kennedy was entirely a domestic plot. No foreign power was involved. While some members of organized crime may have played a contributing role, they were not principals who orchestrated the overthrow of our government in 1963.

CBS News anchor Dan Rather asked me in 1979 if I believed there was a postassassination conspiracy and cover-up by government officials or the Warren Commission to hide the truth regarding the assassination, or were the numerous missteps the result of sheer incompetence.

"I think it was both," I told Mr. Rather. "I think the autopsy and original investigation was sheer incompetency that was in no way meant to be part of a cover-up. I have never suggested that these pathologists or even some members of the Warren Commission knowingly engaged in any kind of a conspiracy. However, I think that as things developed, when they began to realize that there were tremendous defects and gaps in their overall investigation and forensic scientific aspects of the case, they felt that they simply had to put it together in some seemingly plausible scenario. I think it started off as incompetence but that it has become an organized effort to ensure that the truth would never be exposed."[20]

In 1992 Congress passed the JFK Assassination Records Collection Act, which required the establishment of an Assassination Records and Review Board to review and declassify millions of documents related to the president's slaying. Approximately five million such records were made public. It was a huge step forward in discovering what had happened.

While there were no "smoking guns" among the documents, such as the CIA admitting that it was behind the shooting, some records still contained big surprises. For example, there's a previously confidential memo from a lawyer representing Dr. George Burkley, who was President Kennedy's personal physician. Dr. Burkley was present in Dallas when the president was shot. He was present in the emergency room at Parkland Hospital. And he was present during the autopsy. In a 1977 letter to lawyers for the House Select Committee, Dr. Burkley's lawyer stated, "Although he, Burkley, had signed the death certificate of President Kennedy in Dallas, he had never been interviewed and he has information in the Kennedy assassination indicating that others besides Oswald may have participated."[21]

Despite this letter, Dr. Burkley was never officially interviewed by any governmental agency.

The Assassination Records and Review Board also exposed another secret problem: the legitimacy of the autopsy photographs of the brain. During my visit to the National Archives, I noticed that the brain appeared in the photographs to be completely intact. Yet the Zapruder film clearly shows the president's skull exploding, spraying copious amounts of brain matter.

Several witnesses, including a Dallas police officer following the presidential limo, were splattered with brain matter.[22] The chief of anesthesia at Parkland Hospital has stated that, during efforts to resuscitate President Kennedy, Mrs. Kennedy handed him "a large chunk of her husband's brain tissue."[23] In addition, Floyd Riebe, one of the official autopsy photographers, testified that "less than half the brain was there."[24] Shown the official autopsy photographs of the brain that are currently at the National Archives, FBI agent Francis O'Neill, who witnessed the autopsy, claimed that the photographs were inaccurate. "This looks almost like a complete brain," he stated.[25]

The official autopsy report documents the weight of the president's brain to be fifteen hundred grams, which is heavier than the average, complete human brain. In 1998 John Stringer, the lead autopsy photographer, examined the autopsy photographs of President Kennedy's brain. He told the *Washington Post* that the current pictures of the brain are not his and do not resemble anything he saw the night of the autopsy.[26]

Why is this important?

It shows that the Kennedy assassination evidence has been tampered with. Someone does not want the truth to be known. Who that person or those persons are and what their motives may have been, I have no idea.

When I was a young man, I believed that the Kennedy assassination would one day be solved and that the truth would be revealed. As I enter my seventh decade on this Earth, I now have serious doubts. The only way this case will ever be solved is through the reexamination of the physical and medical evidence. Every day that goes by, the evidence deteriorates. If the brain does exist, I doubt it still has any evidentiary value. And I am willing to bet every dollar that I possess that the Kennedy family and the federal government will never allow the body of President Kennedy to be exhumed for a second autopsy.

There was a slight window of opportunity to gain new evidence a few years ago when Governor Connally died. I joined a group of forensic experts and physicians in petitioning then US attorney general Janet Reno to have the bullet fragments removed from the governor's body before he was buried. By obtaining and then testing those bullet fragments, we would have been able to tell for sure if they were fragments from CE 399. Ms. Reno, to our surprise, wrote the Connally family asking for permission to have the bullet fragments surgically removed prior to his burial. However, the family refused, and the bullet fragments, along with possibly our last opportunity for uncovering the truth in the Kennedy assassination, were buried.

Despite my increasing doubt that I will learn the entire truth about the Kennedy assassination in my lifetime, there are legitimate efforts underway that are utilizing advances in science and technology to shed light on the mystery. For example, Dr. Donald Thomas, an expert in the study of acoustical evidence, made a dramatic presentation at a history of the JFK assassination symposium hosted by the Cyril H. Wecht Institute of Forensic Science and Law at Duquesne University in Pittsburgh in November 2003.

As many people may be aware, a Dallas police officer riding a motorcycle accidentally left his microphone on throughout the assassination in Dealey Plaza. As a result, all noises and sounds from the Dealey Plaza area were recorded on a Dallas Police Department Dictaphone. In 1979 the House Select Committee pointed to newly developed acoustical evidence from that recording to reveal that four shots were fired during the attack on President Kennedy.

Using photographs, the Zapruder film, and the Dallas police audio recording, Dr. Thomas's research and analysis, however, showed that there were five shots fired in less than nine seconds. That's right—five shots. At least two of those shots were fired from the grassy knoll area, he explained to the panel. He said a study of the acoustical evidence indicated that the bullets that were fired probably came from a .30-caliber weapon. The most popular and available .30-caliber weapon at that time was a Winchester .30-30 rifle.

Dr. Thomas's findings are quite ironic given the fact that a Dallas police officer based in Dealey Plaza radioed the following alert at 12:45 PM: "The wanted person in this is a slender white male, about thirty, five feet ten, one sixty five, carrying what looked to be a .30-30 or some type of Winchester."[27]

At every turn, the evidence in the Kennedy assassination simply does not add up to a lone gunman. Everywhere I look, the evidence does point to an effort to keep the American public from knowing the truth. Evidence is missing. Witnesses were asked to falsify affidavits. Testimony is dramatically altered. Documents are manipulated.

What happened in Dealey Plaza on November 22, 1963, was an effort by two or more people to kill the president of the United States. What has happened since has been a conspiracy to hide the truth. The result of the two was nothing short of a coup d'état.

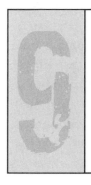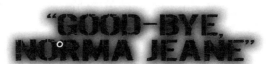

"GOOD-BYE, NORMA JEANE"

THE DEATH OF
MARILYN MONROE

Until his retirement, Dr. Thomas Noguchi was known as "coroner to the stars." Because he served as coroner in Los Angeles, his cases were sometimes high profile, bizarre, and controversial. During his career he performed autopsies on such notables as Natalie Wood, Sharon Tate, William Holden, John Belushi, Janis Joplin, and Robert F. Kennedy. The unparalleled media attention his involvement in such cases would draw made him a near celebrity in Los Angeles County and throughout the country. The popular NBC-TV series *Quincy* was reportedly based on his career. To forensic pathologists worldwide, he is considered one of the best. But to me, Tom has always been a dear friend and respected colleague.

Tom and I had not yet met in the summer of 1962. I finished my forensic pathology fellowship in Baltimore that summer. He earned his medical degree from Nippon Medical School in 1951 and interned at Tokyo University Hospital. After moving to the United States from Japan in 1952, he did a second internship in pathology at Orange County General Hospital, followed by a series of residencies in Los Angeles. We would meet later in February

245

1963 in Chicago at my first conference of the American Academy of Forensic Sciences.

Los Angeles County medical examiner Dr. Theodore J. Curphey hired Tom in 1960 as deputy medical examiner in the coroner's office. Seven years later, Tom was appointed by Los Angeles County officials to replace Dr. Curphey as the chief medical examiner and coroner.

However, on August 5, 1962, that was all yet to be. On that summer day, at about 9:30 AM, Tom strolled into the coroner's office in downtown Los Angeles. On his desk was a note from the coroner's staff: "Dr. Curphey wants Dr. Noguchi to do the autopsy on Marilyn Monroe." He read the investigator's report of a blonde female Caucasian who had been found with empty pill bottles. Included were prescription bottles for Nembutal and chloral hydrate. Dr. Hyman Engelberg, Marilyn's personal physician who pronounced her dead, had prescribed some of the medications. Also in the report was a note: "Psychiatrist talked to her yesterday, very despondent." The thought never occurred to Tom that this could be *the* Marilyn Monroe; he assumed it was a woman with the same name.[1]

As a routine matter, Dr. Noguchi called his boss, Dr. Curphey, to ask if he should go ahead with the autopsy, and he was told to proceed. Tom changed into a plain white cotton autopsy gown with short sleeves, similar to those you see on a supermarket butcher. The gown was county issued, and names were not embroidered or stamped on until the 1980s, when surgical scrubs became popular as outside wear. This was before AIDS, so no masks were required at the time. He was required to wear a full-length vinyl apron that covered his body from neck to shoe top, as well as specially made heavy gloves.

The scenario was a familiar one: the walk down the long corridor on the first floor of the Hall of Justice Building, the scent of formaldehyde, the row of stainless steel tables in the windowless room, the tiled floor. However, the presence of John Miner, deputy district attorney and liaison to the coroner's office, signaled that this was no ordinary case. Dr. Noguchi has said that John Miner was always welcome and that his insights were helpful. However, it should be noted that Miner is not a forensic pathologist and his comments should be taken in that light. He sat in on cases an average of four or five times a year.

As he pulled back the sheet to uncover the body on table 1, he stopped. At that moment, he realized whose autopsy he would be performing that morning and knew that he faced what would become one of the most controversial cases in forensic history.

"I felt a great deal of responsibility," Tom told me later. "I may suppress my emotions, but I am in no way careless or casual about death. My mission was more than curiosity. It was a scientific one."

People have questioned him over and over as to how Marilyn Monroe looked in death, down to details of her manicure. He politely defers an answer to the questions and quotes the Italian poet Petrarch: "It's folly to shrink in fear, if this is dying, for death looked lovely in her lovely face."[2]

From 9:30 AM until about noon, Dr. Noguchi and his technician, Eddy Day, examined the body and performed the autopsy. He started the examination of her body with a handheld magnifying glass, searching for needle marks, which would indicate an injection as well as any other points of trauma. Any good pathologist would do this in a potential drug abuse case. For Dr. Noguchi this painstaking process was customary. "I view the death as a murder until proven otherwise," he told me.

The obvious place for a hard-core addict to shoot up is the antecubital fossa, the front of the elbow. "Cryptic" drug addicts, those who are not out-and-out addicts but who are already in the injection stage of their addiction, tend to shoot up in other places to hide the needle tracks. So pathologists search for marks in remote places—under the finger and toenails, and between the fingers and toes—in short, all over. If a needle site is suspected, an elliptical piece of skin is sliced to see if there is a hemorrhagic track going beneath the epidermis (the outermost layers of the skin). Many things, such as a pimple or a little insect bite, can simulate an injection site, so it is submitted to histology, which is the department responsible for making up microscopic tissue slides. Older needle track marks can be identified but don't tell you anything directly about the death, just about past addiction or injections. Obviously, it is necessary to do this exam first, before the other procedures. Any cutting obscures marks with blood and fluids. On a dark, hairy person, marks are harder to identify. On a fair-skinned person like Marilyn Monroe, they would show up easily. Dr. Noguchi found none.

He noted a slight ecchymotic area, or bruise, approximately two inches in length, which was how he measured bruises at that time, on her lower left back or upper hip on the diagram. Its color, a dark reddish blue, indicated it was a fresh bruise, sustained within a few hours of her death. Not likely caused by violence because of its location and small size, it seemed more consistent with a bump against a table. The rest of his external examination included documenting lividity, which is the settling of the blood from gravity that causes a reddish purple coloration. He also recorded surgical scars and the congestion of conjunctivae, which are the whites of the eyes. This congestion gives the eyes a bloodshot appearance. Except for the bruise on Marilyn's hip, he found no sign of trauma.

Using a scalpel, Dr. Noguchi made the usual Y-shaped incision in the chest cavity. Since he is right-handed, he started from the right shoulder, making an incision to the middle of the chest, and then from the left shoulder to the middle of the chest, forming the top part of the Y. He made a cut downward, thereby exposing the abdomen. He examined her body cavities, cardiovascular system, respiratory system, liver and biliary system, hemic and lymphatic system, digestive system, and urinary system. He observed scar tissue where her gallbladder had been surgically removed, then weighed her heart, lungs, liver, spleen, and kidneys, as well as her brain. Her urine and stomach contents were measured and a gastric smear was made. A pap smear was also taken and her genital system was inspected.

Dr. Noguchi set aside specimens for the toxicology department. Unembalmed blood and the liver would be tested for alcohol and barbiturates. The kidneys, the stomach and its contents, urine, the vaginal smear, and the intestines were also set aside for toxicology. This, by the way, was all contrary to rumors that still surface on the Internet today of her body being embalmed before the autopsy.

Setting aside the intestines is not standard practice. Tom has told me that since he saw no trace of pills in the stomach contents, he wished to utilize the European practice of segmental analysis in which you look at the intestines segmentally to see where the pills are in the intestines and what stages of absorption they are in. This gives a clearer picture of how many pills were taken at one time and how far apart each dosage was, or if they were taken all at once in a massive dose—the single-gulp theory. Dr. Noguchi and his technician were joined by Dr. Curphey at noon and continued the autopsy until about 1:00 PM. The average autopsy usually took Tom about one and a half hours. Marilyn's took three and a half hours.

Following his examination, Dr. Noguchi sat down to his desk and wrote out his report for Marilyn Monroe, Case # 81128, August 5, 1962. The final report was signed on August 27, 1962, as follows. (*I will explain pertinent technical terminology in my summary of the autopsy.*)

> I performed an autopsy on the body of Marilyn Monroe at the Los Angeles County Coroner's Mortuary, Hall of Justice, Los Angeles, and from the anatomic findings and pertinent history I ascribe the death to:
>
> Acute Barbiturate Poisoning
> Due to: Ingestion of Overdose
> (Final 8/27/62)
>
> **ANATOMICAL SUMMARY**

EXTERNAL EXAMINATION:

Lividity of face and chest with a slight ecchymosis of the left side of the back and left hip.

Surgical scar, right upper quadrant of the abdomen.

Suprapubic surgical scar.

RESPIRATORY SYSTEM:

Pulmonary congestion and minimal edema.

LIVER AND BILIARY SYSTEM:

Surgical absence of gallbladder.

Acute passive congestion of liver.

UROGENITAL SYSTEM:

Congestion of kidneys.

DIGESTIVE SYSTEM:

Marked congestion of stomach with petechial mucosal hemorrhage.

Absence of appendix.

Congestion and purplish discoloration of the colon.

EXTERNAL EXAMINATION: The unembalmed body is that of a thirty-six-year-old well-developed, well-nourished Caucasian female weighing 117 pounds and measuring 65½ inches in length. The scalp is covered with bleached blonde hair. The eyes are blue. The fixed lividity is noted in the face, neck, chest, upper portions of the arms, and the right side of the abdomen. The faint lividity which disappears upon pressure is noted in the back and posterior aspect of the arms and legs. A slight ecchymotic area is noted in the left hip and left side of the lower back. The breasts show no significant lesions. There is a horizontal three-inch-long surgical scar in the right upper quadrant of the abdomen. A suprapubic surgical scar measuring five inches in length is noted.

The conjunctivae are markedly congested; however, no ecchymosis or petechiae are noted. The nose shows no evidence of fracture. The external auditory canals are not remarkable. No evidence of trauma is noted in the scalp, forehead, cheeks, lips, or chin. The neck shows no evidence of trauma. Examination of the hands and nails shows no defects. The lower extremities show no evidence of trauma.

BODY CAVITY: The usual Y-shaped incision is made to open the thoracic and abdominal cavities. The pleural and abdominal cavities contain no excess of fluid or blood. The mediastinum shows no shifting or widening. The diaphragm is within normal limits. The lower edge of the liver is within the costal margins. The organs are in normal positions and relationships.

CARDIOVASCULAR: The heart weighs 300 grams. The pericardial cavity contains no excess fluid. The epicardium and pericardium are smooth and glistening. The left ventricular wall measures 1.1 centimeters and the right 0.2 centimeter. The papillary muscles are not hypertrophic. The chordae tendineae are not thickened or shortened. The valves have the usual number of leaflets, which are thin and pliable. The tricuspid valve measures 10 centimeters, the pulmonary valve 6.5 centimeters, the mitral valve 9.5 centimeters, and the aortic valve 7 centimeters in circumference. There is no septal defect. The foramen ovale is closed.

The coronary arteries arise from their usual location and are distributed in normal fashion. Multiple sections of the anterior descending branch of the left coronary artery with a 5-millimeter interval demonstrate a patent lumen throughout. The circumflex branch and the right coronary artery also demonstrate a patent lumen. The pulmonary artery contains no thrombus.

The aorta has a bright yellow smooth intima.

RESPIRATORY SYSTEM: The right lung weighs 465 grams and the left 420 grams. Both lungs are moderately congested with some edema. Edema is bodily fluid outside where it should be; it is fluid without cells. The surface is dark red with mottling. The posterior portion of the lungs shows severe congestion. The tracheobronchial tree contains no aspirated material or blood. Multiple sections of the lungs show congestion and edematous fluid exuding from the cut surface. No consolidation or suppuration is noted. The mucosa of the larynx is grayish white.

LIVER AND BILIARY SYSTEM: The liver weighs 1,890 grams. The surface is dark brown and smooth. There are marked adhesions through the omentum and abdominal wall in the lower portion of the liver, as the gallbladder has been removed. The common duct is widely patent. No calculus or obstructive material is found. Multiple sections of the liver show slight accentuation of the lobular pattern; however, no hemorrhage or tumor is found.

HEMIC AND LYMPHATIC SYSTEM: The spleen weighs 190 grams. The surface is dark red and smooth. Section shows dark red homogeneous firm cut surface. The malpighian bodies are not clearly identified. There is no evidence of lymphadenopathy. The bone marrow is dark red in color.

ENDOCRINE SYSTEM: The adrenal glands have the usual architectural cortex and medulla. The thyroid gland is of normal size, color, and consistency.

URINARY SYSTEM: The kidneys together weigh 350 grams. Their capsules can be stripped without difficulty. Dissection shows a moderately congested parenchyma. The cortical surface is smooth. The pelves and ureters are not dilated or stenosed. The urinary bladder contains approximately 150 cubic centimeters of clear, straw-colored fluid. The mucosa is not altered.

GENITAL SYSTEM: The external genitalia shows no gross abnormality. Distribution of the pubic hair is of female pattern. The uterus is of the usual size. Multiple sections of the uterus show the usual thickness of the uterine wall without tumor nodules. The endometrium is grayish yellow, measuring up to 0.2 centimeter in thickness. No polyp or tumor is found. The cervix is clear, showing no nabithian cysts. The tubes are intact. The openings of the fimbria are patent. The right ovary demonstrates recent corpus luteum haemorrhagicum. The left ovary shows corpora lutea and albicantia. A vaginal smear is taken.

DIGESTIVE SYSTEM: The esophagus has a longitudinal folding mucosa. The stomach is almost completely empty. The content is brownish mucoid fluid. The volume is estimated to be no more than 20 cubic centimeters. No residue of the pills is noted. A smear made from the gastric contents and examined under the polarized microscope shows no refractile crystals. The mucosa shows marked congestion and submucosal petechial hemorrhage diffusely. The duodenum shows no ulcer. The contents of the duodenum is also examined under polarized microscope and shows no refractile crystals. The remainder of the small intestine shows no gross abnormality. The appendix is absent. The colon shows marked congestion and purplish discoloration. The fecal content is light brown and formed. The mucosa shows no discoloration.

The pancreas has a tan lobular architecture. Multiple sections show patent ducts.

SKELETOMUSCULAR SYSTEM: The clavicles, ribs, vertebrae, and pelvic bones show no fracture lines. All bones of the extremities are examined by palpation showing no evidence of fracture.

HEAD AND CENTRAL NERVOUS SYSTEM: The brain weighs 1,440 grams. Upon reflection of the scalp there is no evidence of contusion or hemorrhage. The temporal muscles are intact. Upon removal of the dura mater the cerebrospinal fluid is clear. The superficial vessels are slightly congested. The convolutions of the brain are not flattened. The contour of the brain is not distorted. No blood is found in the epidural, subdural, or subarachnold spaces. Multiple sections of the brain show the usual symmetrical ventricles and basal ganglia. Examination of the cerebellum and brain stem shows no gross abnormality. Following removal of the dura mater from the base of the skull and calvarium, no skull fracture is demonstrated.

Liver temperature taken at 10:30 AM registered 89 degrees F.

SPECIMEN: Unembalmed blood is taken for alcohol and barbiturate examination. Liver, kidney, stomach and contents, urine, and intestines are saved for further toxicological study. A vaginal smear is made.

Dr. Noguchi found no visual evidence of pills in the stomach or the small intestine. According to the reported evidence, she swallowed from twelve to twenty-four Nembutal capsules and enough chloral hydrate capsules to be nearly lethal. Nembutal is a barbiturate and chloral hydrate is a non–barbituric acid derivative. Both are central nervous system depressants that she regularly took as sedatives, or sleeping aids.

His conclusion was that, as a habitual drug user, Marilyn's stomach easily digested the drugs and passed them on into the intestinal tract, much the way a regularly eaten food is digested with less trouble than something new to the system.

Her stomach was almost empty, containing 20 cubic centimeters of brownish mucoid fluid. The fecal contents were formed, inconsistent with a recent enema. There was a purplish discoloration of the colon, which people have made something of, suggesting that it indicated an enema. That's simply not correct at all. This kind of discoloration is common in the postmortem period, especially in people who have been dead for a little bit of time. All the intestinal bacteria become active and the blood begins to settle out. And at her height and weight, she was really quite slender for her build. The more slender the person, the more noticeable the discoloration might be externally.

Because Dr. Curphey knew that signing off the manner of death as "probable suicide" on the death certificate of a world-famous star like Marilyn Monroe was certain to cause controversy, he assembled what would become known as the Suicide Panel. The idea for this panel was later adopted in many instances among professionals throughout the nation. The panel was made up of psychological experts whose job was to interview Marilyn's friends, relatives, and business acquaintances on her psychological makeup, behavior, and background. Confidentiality was promised, and, on Dr. Curphey's orders, the notes were to remain confidential so that individuals involved would speak openly. The fact, however, that the notes have remained closed through the years has almost certainly fueled the rumors of an official cover-up.

In his book, *Coroner*, Dr. Noguchi tells of speaking with one of the panel's founders, Dr. Robert Litman. Dr. Litman, as one of the nation's foremost authorities on suicide, told Tom that he had no doubt that Marilyn had committed suicide.[3]

But let's take a step back. What was it about this girl on table 1 that day that made her so special? Just who was the beauty whose death has evoked such a sense of mystery for more than forty years?

As much as the world feels a personal connection with the star, it is amazing how little accurate information is known about her. Research turns up much that is contradictory, from the spelling of her middle name to when she said what to whom.

She was born Norma Jeane Mortenson on June 1, 1926, at Los Angeles General Hospital to Gladys Monroe Baker. There are doubts as to who her true father was, but he is reported to be Edward Mortenson.[4] He didn't wait around for her birth, so she was later baptized with her mother's last name. The poor girl didn't have a stable childhood. Her clinically depressed mother was said to have had paranoid schizophrenia. Various families cared for Norma Jeane until she was seven, when her mother reclaimed her. Gladys was institutionalized soon after and then married in 1935.[5] Depression seemed to run in the family. Norma Jeane's maternal grandparents also were both rumored to be mentally ill. Della Monroe Grainger and Otis Monroe were both manic-depressive, and Otis reportedly committed suicide. Gladys's grandmother was institutionalized and her great-grandfather purportedly died of psychosis-related causes.

Obviously neither grandparent could offer help in raising their granddaughter. With Gladys unable to effectively care for her daughter, Norma Jeane was raised by a series of foster families, relatives, orphanages, and well-meaning but very strict neighbors. A mainstay foster family was with a friend of her mother's, Grace McKee, who married Ervin Silliman Goddard while the young girl lived there. Norma Jeane was sent away once at age nine to become occupant 3463 at an orphanage and was brought back two years later. It was at her foster home that she would later claim that one of several molestation attempts was made on her as a young-ster. The next would come at the hands of pseudorelatives while living with an uncle's mother.[6]

Marilyn would later say, "The world around me then was kind of grim. I had to learn to pretend in order to . . . I don't know . . . block the grimness. The whole world seemed sort of closed to me. . . . [I felt] on the outside of everything, and all I could do was to dream up any kind of pretend-game."[7]

Whether it was a dream come true or not, she avoided another orphanage at age sixteen when she married her twenty-one-year-old neighbor, Jimmie Dougherty, on June 19, 1942. A picture shows her smiling in a long white wedding dress, beside her new husband, whom she would later call in a letter "just about the greatest man alive." He left Lockheed Aviation two years later to join the Merchant Marines and was sent to Shanghai. She did factory work for Radio Plane Company in Burbank, California.[8] The story could have ended there. Like thousands of other World War II couples, the two could now be celebrating their holidays with great-grandchildren.

But Norma Jeane was discovered by army photographer David Conover at the factory and became a popular cover girl. She had looks and initiative and became a photographer's dream, with her first cover on the January 1946 edition of *Douglas Airview*.[9] She chose her career over marriage and divorced Jimmie in 1946.[10]

"Norma Jeane was always a butterfly," Jimmie Dougherty later wrote in *To Norma Jeane With Love, Jimmie*. "She was beautiful all of her life, within and without. During our courtship and marriage I never stopped loving to be with her, to stare at her, to laugh with and love her. We had a wonderful, joyful marriage. But in the end, it was not enough for Norma Jeane. Like all beautiful butterflies, she had to fly away. . . . I had the honor and privilege to have lived the experience."[11]

She signed her first contract with Fox a few months later for $125 a week. It was then that she bleached her hair and chose her grandmother's last name, becoming the one and only Marilyn Monroe.

Following a series of short-term contracts with different studios and small movie parts, she was soon finding starring roles in movies like *Don't Bother to Knock* and *Niagara.* She made an astonishing thirty movies in fourteen years—comedic hits like *Seven-Year-Itch,* *Gentlemen Prefer Blondes,* and *Some Like It Hot* displaying her talents as an actress and sex symbol.

Her marriages were as famous as her films. When she married Joe DiMaggio, it was one icon joining with another. But that match lasted only nine months. He had a difficult time dealing with having a wife every man wanted. "It's no fun being married to an electric light," the retired Joltin' Joe said.[12]

She later converted to Judaism to marry the great playwright Arthur Miller, first in a civil ceremony and later in a religious one. To some, the match seemed to fit the title of the screenplay he wrote for her, *The Misfits.* But when he was hauled before the House Un-American Activities Committee, she stood by him, and he did his best to help as she battled inner turmoils that no one understood.

"She seemed to have a mind of immense capacity that had been assaulted by life, bludgeoned by a culture that asked only enticement of her," the author wrote of his former wife. "She had acted that role, and was now petitioning for permission to display another dimension."[13] The four-and-a-half-year marriage would end before the film premiered, and Arthur Miller was still a part of her unstable life longer than anyone else.

Whether following her career then or researching her life and death now, Marilyn remains an enigma, a blonde bombshell who studied method acting and had nearly perfect comedic timing. She was perpetually late on the set, but she was a perfectionist about her work. Pills put her to sleep, woke her up, and kept the blues at bay, even as her smile lit up the camera. And nearly everyone interviewed who ever came in contact with her has claimed some sort of intimacy with her. Though much has been rumored about her relationships with the Kennedy brothers, it is impossible to come up with solid documentation of any affair between these very public personages. Her whole life, in fact, seems to dance about, evading recording, with very little there to satisfy the skeptic as being true.

Not long before she died, Richard Merryman, former editor of *Life* magazine, interviewed her. "Her whole reason for being, was the celebrity, by that time. The reason I think she did our piece was that she wanted the reassurance that she was still famous."[14]

Now, more than forty years after her death, she remains an icon like few others. She has been idolized, copied, and imitated, but never replaced. Elton John and Bernie Taupin memorialized her in the song "Candle in the Wind."[15] The US Postal Service placed her image on the thirty-two-cent stamp in 1995.[16] She has been widely impersonated, from Madonna in her "Material Girl" video to tennis star Anna Kournikova in a sportswear ad.[17] A Google search online resulted in approximately 700,000 selections on Marilyn Monroe, 21,210 on simply Norma Jeane, 370 on Norma Jeane Mortenson, 1,500 on Norma Jean Mortenson, 57,540 on Norma Jean Baker, and 1,850 on Norma Jeane Baker.

I learned about Marilyn's death the same way most Americans did—through the newspapers, radio, and television. While the coverage was not as extensive as it would be in today's twenty-four-hour news cycle, the death of such a prominent, beloved, and admired star unquestionably dominated the news.

Beautiful, blonde, sultry—Marilyn portrayed an outward naïveté that made her America's perfect sex symbol. And even though she wasn't my type—I always preferred the cool brunettes like Sophia Loren—I still found her death a tragedy and felt terrible when she died. Whenever a talented person dies—Elvis Presley, Marilyn Monroe, John Belushi, or, in more recent years, John Candy, Selena, or John Ritter—it always seems tragic. Because these people are such wonderful entertainers and should have many more years to bring great pleasure and joy into everyone's lives, we tend to mourn their loss as if they were family. Throughout my career, I've found that to be the case with these tragic deaths of those whose lives end so early and unnecessarily. I remember feeling just that way about Marilyn.

Marilyn's death took hold of the American consciousness. Perhaps it is her fame and charisma that made the public so eager to search for conspiracies. We envy and look up to these stars. A sordid death is not allowed. We demand a beautiful, peaceful death and long life for our "royalty."

In the four decades that followed her untimely demise, Marilyn's death has been engulfed in controversy. In spite of an autopsy that firmly concluded the star had died of an overdose of Nembutal and chloral hydrate, public opinion was determined to find a plot that proved a cause of death other than suicide. So the case was reopened.

There was James Hall, the ambulance attendant, who gave the *Globe* an exclusive interview, stating that he saw a doctor inject something into Marilyn's heart and kill her.[18] Then there was the theory that the actress was drugged at Frank Sinatra's house in Palm Springs and then flown back to her home on 12305 5th Helena Drive in Brentwood, California.[19] Mrs. Murray, Marilyn's housekeeper, came under plenty of suspicion. She was rumored to be on the payroll of Robert Kennedy's brother-in-law, Peter Lawford, to keep quiet about the facts. Some have even accused her of committing the murder herself.[20]

The most popular conjectures seem to involve John and Robert Kennedy and the Mafia. Did Robert Kennedy order the murder to keep Marilyn from going public about her affair with the president? Was the murder planned to keep the public from finding out about Marilyn's pregnancy by one of the two of them, protecting their careers in politics? Did the Mafia order the hit to pay back the US attorney general, their worst enemy, who then raided a Mafia member's home to prevent proof from getting out?

The conspiratorial list of murder suspects by the public became more ludicrous as it grew—the CIA, J. Edgar Hoover, the movie studio, and the doctors. Most of the theories involve death by injection or enema, not pills. Even the FBI had a file on the sexy blonde starlet, with nearly one hundred pages full of inked-out names and activities.

Investigative reporters and conspiracy buffs poured over her short and rather unremarkable autopsy as if they were trained toxicologists. Many were certain that there were clues not yet uncovered or properly scrutinized. Norman Mailer based his biography of Monroe on the theory that the coroner's office wished to find her death to be a suicide.[21]

Questions have arisen on everything about her. Some were legitimate questions to explore. But some were truly preposterous and irrelevant, with unknown origins. She didn't have a sixth toe on one foot, and if she had, it would have had nothing whatsoever to do with her death. In contrast were questions like the following: Why was there no trace of pills in her stomach? Why didn't the yellow dye from the Nembutal, one of the two central nervous system depressants she overdosed on, stain her stomach? Was the bruise on her lower left back an injection site? Was her abdominal scar from a cesarean section? These are understandable questions from a layperson.

I seldom make statements of personal beliefs publicly, preferring to stay within the realm of scientific facts that are laid out in front of me on my table. But from a purely logical point of view, manner of death aside, it simply does not make sense to think that the Kennedy brothers would go through all that trouble, subterfuge, and, most of all, risk, just to silence her at the expense of their political careers. Neither the brothers nor Marilyn was stupid. If affairs did take place, it would certainly seem each one would be smart enough to keep his or her mouth shut. But no matter how preposterous the idea may sound, some people are determined to find a conspiracy in anything.

This is undoubtedly why twenty years after Marilyn's death, on November 4, 1982, Dr. Noguchi found himself in the Criminal Courts Building being questioned by two assistant district attorneys on behalf of the Los Angeles County district attorney's office. Because of the immense public pressure, the case was reopened.

The investigators in the twenty-year-old case concentrated on four main areas:

1. If Marilyn had swallowed the great quantity of pills that were indicated, how could her stomach be empty?
2. Along the same line, why weren't there any partially digested capsules or tablets on the stomach lining? Why didn't the pills leave a powdery residue and possibly cause a raw red appearance on the lining?
3. Why didn't the yellow dye that coated Nembutal stain her stomach?
4. As a matter of their routine practice, Dr. Greenson had given Marilyn Monroe an injection the day before she died. Why didn't Dr. Noguchi find the needle mark?

Dr. Noguchi answered their questions the same way he had answered them in 1962, the same way he answered them for reporters through the years, and the same way he explained them in his best-selling book, *Coroner*.[22] As I have laid out, his findings and beliefs were that the stomach had emptied quickly because it was accustomed to the medication, similar to the stomach's quickly emptying a familiar food. He explained that the petechial hemorrhage, meaning pinpoint, beneath the stomach lining was the raw red appearance that had been caused by the drugs. He called the question regarding Nembutal a layman's question. (As indeed, a medical professional can see that many of the questions regarding Marilyn Monroe are.) The yellow color that coats Nembutal does not run when swallowed. The fourth question was another obvious one for Tom. Dr. Greenson had injected Marilyn forty-eight hours before her death. That would have been made with a fine surgical needle and would have already healed. Dr. Noguchi would most certainly have found any new punctures with his magnifying glass.

A medical examiner from another jurisdiction examined the original autopsy report during the second investigation and also listened to Dr. Noguchi's explanations of details. In December 1982 the Los Angeles district attorney's office released its official report of its investigation into the death of Marilyn Monroe. The report stated the investigators had "uncovered no credible evidence supporting a murder theory."[23]

Dr. Noguchi's professionalism on this case came into question over and over through the years, undoubtedly because of his youth and lack of experience at the time of Marilyn's death. What people didn't seem to realize was that there was a reason that Dr. Curphey had called upon him to do the autopsy. He was the only one on the staff who was a university staff member, holding the position of professor of pathology for Loma Linda University Medical School, and who was board-certified in both clinical and anatomic pathology. He often handled the more difficult scientific cases. Even then, Tom was, quite simply, the most qualified forensic pathologist to conduct the autopsy.

While Tom did not know whether or not Marilyn had affairs with any number of men or who they were, or hold the answers to all the little questions that have nagged through the years, he could answer the mysteries that were solved for him on his autopsy table. A forensic pathologist is given some answers and some clues. There are certain definites in the death of Marilyn Monroe. Still, a few things are subject to a little interpretation. It is here where honest, ethical pathologists can agree to disagree on big cases.

I first became involved in the Marilyn Monroe case later when a variety of journalists began to contact me, asking me for my professional opinion of the autopsy, something that happens quite often in my career. I believe one of the first to get in touch with me was Norman Mailer.

I had been elected in 1969 as coroner of Allegheny County, Pennsylvania, and I was running again four years later in 1973. Mailer was very gracious and agreed to be my guest of honor for a fund-raising event. We spent the day together discussing the fund-raiser and my interpretation of the autopsy as he prepared to write what would be considered his somewhat speculative biography, *Marilyn*.[24]

I remember that Vice President Spiro Agnew had just resigned on October 10 and pleaded no contest to a charge of federal income tax evasion. In his inimitable style, Mailer spoke extemporaneously at the fund-raiser and discussed the resignation and the subsequent selection of Gerald Ford as Agnew's replacement. It was a very interesting commentary on a significant moment in US history.

Subsequently, he cordially invited my wife, Sigrid, and me to his lovely home in Brooklyn Heights, New York, a very nice residential area. We walked in and met some celebrities and authors, including Daniel Ellsberg, who had leaked the Pentagon Papers, and the best-selling author E. L. Doctorow, who had just written *Book of Daniel* and would soon publish *Ragtime*.

By that time, I had received a copy of the autopsy report and had plenty of information on hand to use in dealing with Mailer as well as members of the media. I was subsequently contacted by other authors and have been on a variety of talk shows and news programs regarding this case.

Most of the cases I handle outside of my capacity as coroner come to me through attorneys who hire me as an expert or independent forensic pathologist. Sometimes the family of the victim or defendant may consult me directly. Of course, consultations with attorneys are official, and I charge for them. At other times the news media will contact me. I don't consider those formal consultations, and I never charge for those. I'll get a call from TV, radio, or newspapers anywhere in the country. I'll have all kinds of inquiries and requests, often after reviewing the autopsy report.

Some of the inquiries refer to very interesting cases. And that is how I got involved with the case of Marilyn.

When I am asked to review someone's autopsy, famous or otherwise, I analyze it step by step, as if I were actually performing the autopsy myself. I pay particular attention to the sections that I know are under question. And that is exactly what I did in this case.

The nude body of Marilyn Monroe was found lying facedown on her bed. At five feet five and a half inches and 117 pounds, her petite body was quite curvaceous. The dressmaker gave her measurements as 36-22-36. All these statistics and the gowns she left behind argue against the assumption that Marilyn was "full figured" by today's standards.

Dr. Noguchi found fixed lividity in the face, neck, chest, upper portions of the arms, and the right side of the abdomen, which was consistent with the prone position that her body was found lying in. There was a faint lividity in the back and posterior aspect of the arms and legs that disappeared with faint pressure. It should be noted here that to the untrained eye lividity is often misinterpreted as bruising because the discoloration is the same. A bruise is caused by blood that has escaped from damaged blood vessels. Lividity is from blood still inside engorged blood vessels. So what some laypeople have thought to be bruising on the backs of Marilyn's arms and legs was, in actuality, lividity. Except in certain cases, such as carbon monoxide poisoning, where it is pinkish red, lividity is usually dusky purplish red, a bluish red. Lividity, also known as livor mortis, indicates the position of the body after death. It does not tell the cause of death or the manner of death. Livor mortis, which becomes apparent thirty minutes to two hours after death, is the settling of the blood as the result of gravity.

Rigor mortis is different. Rigor mortis is the stiffening of the body after death because of the disappearance of adenosine triphosphate (ATP) from the muscle. ATP is the basic source of energy for muscle contraction, and none is produced after death.

Violent muscular exertion brings on a decrease of ATP. If this violent exercise or exertion occurs immediately before death, it can speed up rigor mortis. Sometimes, in such instances, it can begin in minutes. Otherwise, rigor mortis usually begins to appear two to four hours after death and disappears with decomposition. The development of rigor mortis varies greatly depending on body temperature, weather, heavy exercise, convulsions, and even manner of death. Because of the varying factors, neither rigor mortis nor livor mortis is entirely reliable for pinpointing time of death. Both, however, can indicate whether the body has been moved.

Conspiracy theorists use the faint secondary lividity on the back and posterior of the arms and legs to argue that the body was moved. The body was found facedown. Since officials were not called in until 4:25 AM, she had been dead long enough to develop livor mortis of the face, neck, chest, upper portions of the arms, and right side of the abdomen. In America bodies are too often laid on their backs on the stretchers for transport. This causes a secondary lividity. Coroners need the bodies transported to the morgue in as close to the same position as they are found or else misleading interpretations can be made. Instead, we must often talk to the ambulance drivers to find the initial position of the body. The reasoning for this change in position comes from our widespread practice of open-casket funerals. A body left on its face too long will develop such intense livor mortis that the funeral home will not be able to disguise it properly. This is not a situation that makes coroners happy, but it is one that, for the present, as forensic pathologists, we must work around.

Ecchymosis, or the discolored area found on Marilyn's left hip and the left side of her lower back, is simply another word for bruise or contusion. It should be noted that Dr. Noguchi describes this in the singular fashion, as one bruise. Laypeople often think the explanation of the area, "the left side of the back *and* left hip," means more than one bruise, whereas it is actually a description of the location of the bruise. The color, a dark reddish blue, indicated a fresh bruise about two inches long that was only a few minutes to a few hours old. Bruises become more prominent after a person has been dead awhile. Bruises occur when tiny blood vessels are broken from an external trauma. Breakdown of the red blood cells causes the bruise to change color in stages—from dark reddish blue or purple to orangish brown, then yellowish brown, and then to the green and yellow one sees right before a bruise heals. In fact, in some places in England, if the coroner has a body that he thinks has been injured or beaten, he lets the body lie for a day or two. As noted, this allows the discoloration to become more prominent.

It is often conjectured that Marilyn's bruise was caused by a fatal injection in the hip, producing death by drug overdose, while making it look like a suicide. This speculation is based on people's experiences with having blood taken by an intravenous puncture. When the needle does not go directly into the vein or pressure is not properly applied as the needle is withdrawn, the blood seeps out, and many people get some bruising. But with a hip injection, there is no bruising. The discoloration is due to seepage of blood. Seepage of blood is due to perforation of a vein by a needle, and there are no blood vessels damaged when you stick a needle into fatty tissue.

To accept this discolored area on Marilyn's hip as just a bruise from a bump or a fall is no great stretch. In fact, the stretch would be to say that it came from a needle. She was a fair-skinned woman with drugs in her system. Her light complexion would not only cause her to bruise easily, but would also make any needle mark readily apparent. At five feet five and a half inches in height, her hip was level with tabletops. She could very easily have bumped into something and sustained a bruise.

Marilyn's three-inch and five-inch surgical scars were attributable to her missing gallbladder and appendix. The three-inch-long horizontal scar in the right upper quadrant of the abdomen was from gallbladder surgery. Her appendectomy, like the gallbladder surgery, was, of course, not at that time done laparoscopically. It still was not a classic appendectomy scar, but rather a suprapubic one. She probably wanted the five-inch-long scar below her "bikini line" so that it would not show in photo shoots. Questions have been raised as to whether it was from a past cesarean section, but it was not a typical C-section scar. And there is also the fact that her appendix was absent.

Dr. Noguchi noted marked congestion of the conjunctivae: this is the whites of the eyes, and the congestion is simply a result of her being in a prone position when she died. Congestion means that the blood vessels are engorged, whether they are arteries, veins, small arterioles, venules, or capillaries. It is just a matter of gravity with the very tiny capillaries and the conjunctivae becoming engorged. A hemorrhage is different. Hemorrhage is blood outside the vessels. When it occurs in the conjunctivae, it is called a *petechial* hemorrhage, Latin for pinpoint, and it gives the eyes a bloodshot appearance. We look for this as evidence of a strangling. There was no ecchymosis or petechial hemorrhaging of the whites of her eyes. They were congested, and I would expect that in someone lying facedown.

The next point in the autopsy consists only of six sentences. Little has been made of this point, but it says quite a lot in this particular case:

> The nose shows no evidence of fracture. The external auditory canals are not remarkable. No evidence of trauma is noted in the scalp, forehead, cheeks, lips, or chin. The neck shows no evidence of trauma. Examination of the hands and nails shows no defects. The lower extremities show no evidence of trauma.

If we address this from the perspective of Marilyn as a potential murder victim, trauma is an important aspect. In a homicide of this nature, one would expect some evidence of a conscious struggle. No one is going to be able to give an individual a forceful enema, as has been speculated, without a struggle. A forensic pathologist would expect to find some injuries on the victim of such a scenario.

There was no evidence of trauma to the nose or ears. Dr. Noguchi told me that he examined her scalp with his magnifying glass, as well as her forehead, cheeks, lips, and chin. There were no injuries. The same kind of examination revealed no evidence of trauma to her neck, hands, or nails. He also examined the lower half of her body with his magnifying glass and found no signs of trauma. If a person bumps his head on a cabinet, it shows up in an autopsy. The only place on Marilyn's body showing any trauma was the bruise on her hip.

Trauma can mean any type of cut, scrape, bruise, or even any internal injury. Unless she was incapacitated in some way, there would be some evidence of bruising on her hands, shoulders, elbows, or hips—all dependent on how she was being held down. But if she were being given a forceful enema or injection without the means of sedation, there would be signs of trauma.

Everything in the pleural and abdominal cavities appeared normal, with no excess fluid or blood. There was no shifting or widening of the mediastinum, the space in the middle of the chest. The organs were in place, and the liver was not enlarged. This is demonstrated by the fact that the lower edge of the liver was within the costal region, or did not extend below the bottom of the rib cage. So even though Marilyn liked her cocktails, her liver did not appear to be damaged. Pills do not enlarge the liver.

Dr. Noguchi's assessment of the cardiovascular system also showed no abnormalities. The heart weighed 300 grams and was perfectly healthy. She had no coronary artery disease, congenital anomalies, acquired cardiac problems, or blood clots. "Patent lumen" is a term used often in the autopsy. *Patent* means it is normal and *lumen* is the opening of a vessel, so it simply means the vessel opening is normal.

Inspection of the lungs showed no signs of pneumonia and made it clear that she had not vomited. There was some moderate congestion with edema, and the posterior portions displayed severe congestion. This means that the lungs contained fluid, called pulmonary edema. An abnormal finding, we often see this in someone who dies of a drug overdose. The brain becomes clinically depressed by the medications. In turn, it depresses the heart and lung functions. When the heart is depressed, it doesn't beat effectively, so blood backs up and fluid escapes into the lungs. Then we have pulmonary congestion. Everything becomes so congested that the fluid part of the blood escapes from the tiny capillaries in the lungs and produces pulmonary edema—fluid in the alveoli, or air sacs.

It is a rather vicious cycle because the lungs are already functioning inadequately because of the depressed control mechanism from the brain. When Marilyn overdosed, her breathing was compromised. That is part of the terminal process. Her heart began to fail. Congestion of her lungs increased, and the pulmonary fluid continued to build up. The aeration process became further compromised as the drugs continued to depress her brain. As the fluid accumulated, oxygenation was diminished.

Oxygenation takes place at the air sac level. Each air sac is called an alveolus; there are hundreds of thousands of these alveoli. Microscopically, the lining of each air sac is an alveolar capillary, and that is where the blood/gas exchange takes place. The lungs give off carbon dioxide and oxygen is picked up. When these air sacs fill with fluid, obviously, there cannot be a proper blood/gas exchange. So oxygenation is diminished. And the vicious cycle continues.

When someone dies of a drug overdose, she doesn't die in a second. It could be minutes. It could be hours. This process usually develops very slowly and insidiously and worsens as the victim becomes unconscious. Marilyn began to gasp for breath, but not in the way that someone short of breath would. And because pulmonary edema usually develops more slowly in drug overdose cases, Marilyn probably did not choke. That occurs when the fluids build up rapidly. With overdose cases, there is continuing diminution of consciousness, and so, as Marilyn became slowly unconscious, she probably was not really gasping heavily for breath or even choking in the way one sees dramatized. After a while, as her lungs ceased to function properly, her breathing became noisy, shallow, and weak. She probably did not even realize what was happening by that time.

Because of the congestion, the liver was rather heavy at 1,890 grams. The congestion came from the backup of blood. Again, this was brought about by the failure of the heart to beat effectively. The lobular pattern on the liver is congestion of the liver brought on by drug death. The spleen was enlarged and congested as well at 190 grams. Her combined kidney weight was normal at 350 grams. Dissection of the kidneys showed a congested parenchyma. The "parenchyma" is the functioning part of any organ. The bladder held a little more than five ounces, or 150 cubic centimeters, of urine.

The description of the ovaries indicates all was normal. The recent corpus luteum haemorrhagicum in the right ovary and the corpora lutea and albicantia in the left ovary simply mean she had just menstruated. Much speculation has been engaged in over the years about Marilyn's supposed pregnancies, miscarriages, and abortions. This is an area where forensic medicine has its limits. Sometimes the cervix will show whether or not someone has been pregnant before, but it still remains questionable. An exam usually doesn't show prior pregnancies that have aborted or miscarried early. However, most of the time doctors can tell if someone has actually given birth to a baby. It has to do with what happens to the cervix, the lower uterine segment. Since prior full-term pregnancies were not indicated in Marilyn's autopsy, we must assume there were none.

With only 20 cubic centimeters, or less than one ounce, of fluid in the stomach, Marilyn had no food in her system to help delay absorption of the drugs. This enabled the normal gastric juices to get to work on the drugs quickly and directly. This helps to explain the lack of pills or residue in her stomach. Nembutal and chloral hydrate are fast-acting drugs by nature anyway, and the lack of food helped to speed their path to the beginning of the small intestine. Much has also been made of the lack of any refractile crystals from the drugs. They left no crystal residue. This does not indicate an enema as some suppose, since we don't necessarily find crystalline material with these drugs. Absorption of the Nembutal and chloral hydrate took place rapidly, in less than an hour. It takes a while for the drugs to get into the blood and affect the brain, and, as I said, she probably did not die immediately, but lingered on, moving from an unconscious state into a deeper stupor, into a coma, and then death.

The inner lining of the stomach, called the mucosa, was congested. The submucosa, which lies just beneath it, showed diffuse petechial hemorrhages. In my opinion, this simply means that drugs were present in the stomach and caused superficial irritation. If something irritates the stomach lining, it can cause actual hemorrhages. A minor irritant or overall congestion can cause pinpoint hemorrhaging.

The reddish purplish discoloration of the colon that is mentioned has nothing to do with an enema. I see this quite frequently in postmortem examinations. It has no significance in this particular case, either. Dr. Noguchi told me later that he found the fecal contents to be normally formed and more consistent with regular bowels than that of someone who had been given an enema.

There was no evidence of fractures. This is another negative finding arguing against a very rough manhandling. If Marilyn was drugged and then murdered, there would not be any fractures. However, fractures might have occurred if she was fighting back.

The brain was swollen and a little heavy, weighing 1,440 grams. This is in line with what we often see in a drug death. Again, she had congestion in the superficial vessels, or small arteries and veins overlying the surface of the brain. Everything else was normal. Even forty years ago, just a small bump on the head would have been found in a thorough autopsy like this one.

And there were no signs of head trauma. This would be entirely consistent with the type of woman who stayed at home in her robe a good deal of the time, chatting on the phone with friends. It would not be consistent with someone who had been forcibly drugged.

The liver temperature specifies algor mortis, the postmortem body temperature, which is taken to help indicate time of death. It was taken at 10:30 AM and registered at 89 degrees F. The body loses one and a half to two degrees the first hour and one degree each hour thereafter. A special thermometer is inserted deep into the rectum or into the liver at the scene of death. Since the body had been refrigerated at the medical examiner's office, algor mortis cannot be applied and would not have had any relevance in this case. This is one more instance of how vital it is in investigations for bodies to be properly handled after death.

When Marilyn was found dead on her bed on August 5, 1962, the prescription bottles that had taken over her life and eventually helped to end it surrounded her. The toxicology laboratory of the Los Angeles County coroner listed the following prescriptions in the "Report of Chemical Analysis":

Prescription #19295: Filled on 06/07/62 for Librium; 5 mgm; 50 capsules. Found with 27 remaining.

Prescription #20201: Filled on 07/10/62 for Librium; 10 mgm; 100 capsules. Found with 17 capsules remaining.

Prescription #20569: Filled on 07/25/62 for Sulfathalli-dine; 36 tablets. Found with 26 remaining.

Prescription #20858: Filled on 08/03/62 for Nembutal (pentobarbital); 1½ gr (100 mg); 25 capsules. Found empty.

Prescription #20570: Filled on 07/25/62 for chloral hydrate; 0.5 gm (500 mg); 50 capsules. Refilled on 7/31/62. Found with 10 capsules remaining.

Prescription #456099: Filled on 11/04/61 for Noludar; 50 capsules. Found empty.

32 peach-colored tablets marked MSD in prescription-type vial without label.

Prescription #20857: Filled on 08/03/62 for Phenergan; 25 mg; 25 pills.

Chloral hydrate is a central nervous system depressant that was once used a great deal more than it is today. It is a sedative and a non–barbituric acid derivative. When used as a sleep aid or a procedural or postoperative sedative, the recommended oral dose for adults is 0.5 gram (gm) to 1.0 gram. This should not exceed 2 grams in twenty-four hours and is only meant for short-term use, since it may be habit forming. The prescription bottle, number 20570, which was found by Marilyn's bed, was filled on July 25, 1962, and originally contained fifty chloral hydrate capsules at 0.5 gram.

The blood level for chloral hydrate in her toxicology report was 8.0 milligrams percent. This is very, very high. A blood level as low as 1.0 milligram percent can sometimes cause death. Considering the earlier prescription and the refill just four days earlier, with only ten capsules left, we can estimate her usage at an average of approximately ten capsules per day. Maximum recommended daily intake at her dosage (0.5 gm) was four capsules per day. This equals the maximum allowable 2 grams per twenty-four hours. With ten 0.5-gram capsules per day, she was taking 5.0 grams (5,000 mg) per day. She may have developed somewhat of a tolerance, but this level of chloral hydrate combined with the high level of pentobarbital would definitely have been lethal. Her blood concentration level at death was consistent with her consuming five 0.5-gram capsules, or 2.5 grams of chloral hydrate. We can estimate the dose based upon the blood level concentration.

Nembutal is a fast-acting barbiturate. It was the only barbiturate found that was available to Marilyn. Because of this, we know that the barbiturate level in her blood of 4.5 milligrams percent listed in the toxicology report was pentobarbital, or

Nembutal. The liver pentobarbital concentration was 13.0 milligrams percent.

We can use the distribution pattern and the blood concentration level to estimate the dose of Nembutal as well. We know the peak serum concentration following a single oral 100-milligram (1½ grains) dose of Nembutal. Marilyn Monroe had her prescription for twenty-five 100-milligram capsules of Nembutal filled on August 3, two days before her death. Judging by the fact that the bottle was empty, correlated with the toxic levels in her liver and blood, we can estimate that she took between twelve and twenty-four capsules. It is much more likely that she took closer to twenty-four capsules.

Since both pentobarbital (Nembutal) and chloral hydrate are central nervous system depressants, taking them together in these amounts creates a lethal additive effect. While her likely tolerance for chloral hydrate may have saved her life from the ingestion of that drug alone—an amount that would kill most people—the combination would certainly be fatal.

Judging by the dates the prescriptions were filled and the number of remaining capsules, we can estimate that Marilyn was also taking three to four 10-milligram capsules of Librium a day, which is within the recommended daily dose for mild anxiety disorders. Her prescription for one hundred 10-milligram capsules of Librium was filled on July 10, and there were seventeen left at the time of her death. However, she also had a prescription for fifty 5-milligram capsules filled earlier, on June 7. Since she had twenty-seven capsules left, it doesn't appear that she took them on a regular basis. Accurate estimated dosage isn't possible. She probably didn't take Nembutal or chloral hydrate during the daytime; Librium was probably the drug that she took to help her make it through the day. It takes several hours for peak blood levels to be reached, and the half-life of the drug is at the very least twenty-four hours. Since there was no trace of any found in her blood, it is reasonable to assume that either she had taken none that Saturday or had taken it so close to the time of her death that it did not show up in the results.

The earlier prescription for Noludar, a type of sedative, filled in November 1961, was not likely involved in her death. Sulfathallidine is one of the sulfa drugs, which is usually used for urinary tract infections. As a note of interest, she was taking these exactly as prescribed, possibly to clear up an infection. But she died with twenty-six pills left. The peach-colored tablets marked MSD in the unlabeled container appear to be consistent with a diuretic (hydrodiuril) marketed by Merck Pharmaceutical. Phenergan is an antiallergic and is often used as a cold medication or sedative. None of these medications is likely to have played a role in her death.

Phenobarbital was absent, and the test for alcohol came up negative.

Much argument has been made over Marilyn's empty stomach. It has been the basic crux of the murder theory. I just don't see any problem with the fact that the drugs were not there. Again, when we have a stomach free of food, the drugs are going to be absorbed more rapidly into the system.

Marilyn died of lethal amounts of Nembutal and chloral hydrate. "Cause of death" is literally what causes you to die. Marilyn Monroe's cause of death was acute barbiturate poisoning. The main question in this death, however, was not the cause of death, but the manner of death. Dr. Noguchi had listed, and Dr. Curphey had signed off on, "probable suicide" as the manner of death.

Actually, this is rather unusual. The manner of death, in decreasing order of occurrence, is: natural, accident, suicide, or homicide. That is the manner of death. I would infer that because she was Marilyn Monroe and because of the pressures from Hollywood and celebrities, Dr. Curphey and Dr. Noguchi added the word "probable." If it had been Susie Jones or Mary Smith, it would have been termed a suicide. In other words, the word "probable" was there to allow all the Hollywood devotees to think, "Gee, maybe she didn't really commit suicide. Marilyn's autopsy says 'probable.' It doesn't say 'definite,' or simply 'suicide.'"

On a death certificate from a coroner/medical examiner's office, we do not enter "probable." If we don't know how the person died, we put "undetermined," which is another category for the manner of death available to coroners and medical examiners. It is not available to doctors in hospitals, however. The only manner of death allowed for doctors in hospitals to list is "natural." Homicides, suicides, accidents—any unnatural death—must be handled by the coroner or medical examiner. It is infrequent, but not at all rare, that medical examiners and coroners list the manner of death as "undetermined." Perhaps that is what the medical examiner's office in Los Angeles should have done in this case, if they were truly uncertain.

A good example would be when someone is found dead in the car in his garage. The body has a high carbon monoxide level, but there is no hose attachment or suicide note. He had been drinking. What do I know for certain? Maybe he intended to commit suicide. Maybe he came home drunk and thought he'd sleep it off in the car and didn't want to wake up his wife. So in a case like that I might list the manner of death as undetermined. The cause of death would clearly be carbon monoxide poisoning. When a coroner can't make a definite decision based on scientific and investigative facts it should be left as undetermined. A final decision doesn't need to be made immediately. "Probable" is a fine assumption to begin with, but there is no place on the death certificate for the words "probable," "possible," "most likely," "very likely," or "slightly likely." The coroner just doesn't get into that.

Another term we don't use is "accidental suicide." Accidental suicide is an oxymoron. Some people talk about automatism—the idea that when the drug is taken, it has an effect on the central nervous system and the victim becomes confused. We theorize that can happen. For example, some sedatives, instead of having a sedating effect, may cause people to behave bizarrely or become confused and forget they took the drug. Then they take some more. They forget again and take even more.

If you don't intend to kill yourself, then it is an accident. If you believe in the phenomenon of automatism, then it is not a suicide. It is an accident.

An interesting case scenario showing the difference between an accidental ingestion of a lethal amount of drugs or alcohol and suicide by means of overdose is in the autopsy of Elvis Presley. I reviewed his autopsy for the ABC News program *20/20*. When Elvis died, he had twelve central nervous system depressants in his system.[25] Marilyn Monroe had two. When the decedent has taken so much of one drug that it is enough to cause death by itself, the most likely explanation is suicide, unless there is some reasonable theory or basis to infer that the person took the drug unwittingly. The number of prescription analgesics, sedatives, and tranquilizers in Elvis's system was clearly indicative of an accidental overdose. Because of the various levels of each prescription medication in his blood, it can be assumed that Elvis was taking them without real- izing the potential inherent dangers in combining them.

Some people abuse drugs and die from it. Herein lies the great danger of any type of abuse. Unpredictably and inexplicably, there may be a serious adverse effect. Why did it not happen the previous time when they used the same amount of drugs? We don't know the answer to that. It is not always dose related. Sometimes a drug can trigger a cardiac arrhythmia and the person goes on to die because he does not have cardiorespiratory resuscitation. Nobody is around to help, or friends panic and don't want to call 911 for fear of getting themselves in trouble with the cops for being involved with illicit drugs.

These are accidental deaths. So we don't designate them as sui- cides. In spite of the deliberate ingestion or injection, the death is an accident. They are drug abuser deaths—mostly from heroin. Nowadays, Oxycontin is a popular painkiller. Sometimes known as oxycodone, it is in the codeine family and is a big drug of abuse, both by prescription and on the streets. This is the drug allegedly abused by Rush Limbaugh.[26]

With Marilyn Monroe we know there was a large amount of barbiturates in her system. Because of this, some begin to speculate on how the drugs got there and whether somebody came in and gave her an enema or injection.

The truth about Marilyn's death, however, is that, no matter how dramatic, mysterious, or conspiratorial people try to make it, everything indicates that she overdosed, be it deliberately or by accident, on Nembutal and chloral hydrate. They were both pre-scribed central nervous system depressants typically used for sleep aids. Chloral hydrate is also a prime ingredient in the well-known Mickey Finn. By simply judging the scientific evidence left by her own body, which is what I do, I find no verification of foul play. In fact, the more I examine the issues, the more evidence I see that points to suicide.

The fact that the toxicology department disposed of all but the blood and the liver adds to the dispute over Marilyn's death. This doesn't mean that the head toxicologist, Raymond J. Abernathy, deliberately ordered the specimens destroyed. Abernathy told Noguchi that he disposed of all the other organs because the case had been closed. But I am certain that Mrs. John Doe would not be treated the same as a star. It was surely all over the department that it was Marilyn Monroe's intestines they were handling. I don't think it was a calculated cover-up, but the toxicologist certainly doesn't get a free ride here.

I have trusted Tom Noguchi for many years, both as a friend and as a forensic pathologist. Up until the day he retired, he was one of the best coroners and medical examiners in the country. He is also trustworthy and honorable. The rumors that have spread regarding any type of a cover-up on his part are impossible for me to believe. After separating scanty facts from numerous rumors, little is left for us to consider scientifically but the autopsy. If I did not trust the coroner, I would experience natural skepticism here, and, of course, as a scientist I always double-check everyone. But I cannot say this with any more authority: I trust Dr. Noguchi's ethics and professionalism. Tom would never be part of a conspiracy or cover-up. It is simply not part of his moral fiber.

Much has been said of Marilyn's state of mind the few weeks before she died. Twentieth-Century Fox was reportedly opening talks of bringing her back so they could resume shooting on *Something's Got to Give,* the picture she had been fired from for continual tardiness and refusal to show up for work. Talks were also in the works for a Broadway musical and a Las Vegas show. She supposedly was on very good terms with Joe DiMaggio again, and discussions of remarrying were taking place. On the other hand, if rumors are correct, her relationship with the Kennedys was on the downside and her phone calls were no longer being returned.

Dr. Ralph Greenson, her nearly full-time psychiatrist, had her hire Eunice K. Murray to keep house and look out for her. Dr. Greenson and Dr. Hyman Engelberg were supposed to be working together to reduce the number and amount of sedatives Marilyn took and to insure they did not unwittingly double up on their prescriptions. Judging by the medications found at her death, they were not always successful in this venture.

Like thousands of women across America that morning, Marilyn Monroe had orange juice for breakfast on August 4, 1962. She sat at the table in a blue robe and seemed unusually cheerful to the housekeeper. Then she asked an odd question. She wanted to know if there was any oxygen in the house, to which Mrs. Murray said no. Since Marilyn didn't have any breathing problems, Mrs. Murray became so concerned that she called Dr. Greenson. He came later and spent a couple of hours with Marilyn, but he never explained why she had wanted the oxygen. We don't know what this question indicates. One can only speculate whether the star already had intentional overdose and possible resuscitation on her mind. Perhaps she was making sure nothing was around for that resuscitation or, conversely, that it would be possible. We know only that she told Mrs. Murray that she was "just curious." She had attempted suicide before but always only to a point at which she could be rescued.

Marilyn spent most of the day in her robe, sitting in bed and talking on the phone at her Spanish Colonial hacienda. Ironically, the Latin engraving at the door read "Cursum Perficio," meaning "My journey ends here." This was a normal thing for her, and her mood still seemed fine to the housekeeper. About 7:30 PM she had what seemed to be an enjoyable conversation with Joe DiMaggio Jr., her ex-husband's son. Another conversation, just thirty minutes later, was with the actor Peter Lawford, brother-in-law to President Kennedy. Her slightly slurred last words to him at about 8 PM are probably the last words anyone heard her say. She let him know she couldn't join him with friends for a poker game and dinner, and then she said, "Say good-bye to Pat [Patricia Kennedy Lawford], say good-bye to the President. Say good-bye to yourself because you've been a good guy." That was all.

As noted before, Marilyn's empty stomach caused the large amounts of drugs she took to start acting immediately. It would appear that she took the overdose sometime between her conversation with Joe DiMaggio Jr. at 7:30 PM and her 8 PM conversation with Peter Lawford. The vicious cycle we have described is a varying one. But because of the fast-acting nature of the drugs, the large dosage she consumed, and the lack of food to absorb them, the spiraling cycle was speeded up. It can be calculated that Marilyn Monroe was dead by 9 or 9:30 PM.

Since no one else heard from Marilyn Monroe again, the rest is pieces of facts many have attested to as "eyewitness." The running joke is that if everyone was at Marilyn Monroe's house that night of her death who claimed to be, or who was supposedly spotted there, they would have spilled into the streets. For this reason, as happens in many well-known cases, the timeline following her death requires a bit of conjecture.

Marilyn's slurred usage of the word "good-bye" worried Lawford, so he called his manager, who reportedly told him that, as a relative of the president, he couldn't possibly check on Marilyn Monroe in person. More calls were made by Lawford and then by others, and, amazingly, none of them to any type of officials. Marilyn's agent, Milton Rudin, called her about 9:30 PM to check on her. Mrs. Murray told Rudin that her light was on and the telephone cord was under the door. Evidently this reassured Rudin, and Mrs. Murray went to sleep. She woke up later to find Marilyn's light still on and her door locked. She called Dr. Greenson, who broke into the room from the outside window with a fireplace poker. Apparently, phoning the fire department, ambulance, or police didn't enter anyone's mind.

Dr. Greenson finally called the police at 4:25 AM, Sunday, August 5. Sgt. Jack Clemons logged the call. Thinking it a prank, he drove over by himself instead of sending a squad car. Mrs. Murray told him they had found the body around midnight. Dr. Greenson explained that they had been calling the studio and her business associates. Of course, the officer couldn't help but wonder why these calls had taken four hours. Today, this time period plays a great part in the conspiracy theories surrounding the death of Marilyn Monroe.

I do not know why Dr. Greenson chose to call Hollywood acquaintances before calling authorities, as he properly should have. This probably had to do with trying to protect her celebrity status. If and why Mrs. Murray was washing sheets hasn't been answered in more than forty years and probably never will be, neither will many other issues that have been rumored. We do know that eyewitnesses are seldom as reliable as they think they are and twenty witnesses to a head-on collision often report seeing twenty different things. However, none of this affects the results of the autopsy. The dead may not speak, but they do not tell lies. And the rumors are silenced when science does its work.

"Do you remember when Marilyn Monroe died?" Marlon Brando once asked. "Everybody stopped work, and you could see all that day the same expressions on their faces, the same thought: 'How can a girl with success, fame, youth, money, beauty . . . how could she kill herself?' Nobody could understand it because those are the things that everybody wants, and they can't believe that life wasn't important to Marilyn Monroe, or that her life was elsewhere."[27]

The important thing to remember here is that you cannot think rationally and get into the mind of someone who commits suicide. When trying to be rational in approach, we cannot understand someone who is feeling self-disgust, self-loathing, or severe depression. For whatever reason, a suicidal person believes she has not measured up to a self-set level and worries about disappointing friends, family, and loved ones. Feeling ashamed or embarrassed, she may feel completely abandoned or shunned.

When we discuss possible suicide cases—for example, the musician Kurt Cobain who died just over ten years ago—we cannot just examine simple surrounding circumstances when deciding on a verdict of suicide or homicide. Suicidal people are not rational and do not address problems the way rational thinkers do. As a forensic pathologist, I can look at the whole picture, including a person's background, but must rely on science and the body on the table in front of me to show the way and provide the answers.

In many of the cases in which people, usually young men, hang themselves in jail, the incarceration is not for a major crime. To the average person these crimes—public nuisance, drunk driving, domestic violence—would appear to be an absurd reason to commit a slow, painful suicide by hanging. Murderers, armed robbers, or rapists don't usually hang themselves. Jail hangings are usually associated with those who commit minor crimes. They're not monsters. They're not psychopaths. They're ashamed. They're embarrassed. Their psyche is such at the time that they cannot logically think of another option.

That is why the suicide rate is relatively low—most people have the psychological ability to rationalize and explain things to themselves. If not, many more people would be committing suicide. We handle our guilt; we adjust, accommodate, and rationalize. Sometimes we delude ourselves too much. However, some people don't have that psychogymnastic ability to nimbly bounce guilt or depression around in their brains. They just become dejected and despondent. As to determining whether or not a death was a suicide by examining their reason to live, I'm not saying that a reason to live is not a factor to consider—it is. I'm saying in and of itself, it is not a determinant. You can't tell whether someone had a lot to live for despite some setbacks. Ninety-nine percent of the people out there may be able to deal with a bad situation, but there is the 1 percent who can't and who commits suicide.

In Marilyn's case, many people reject the possibility of suicide out of hand, because she seemed to have it all. She was beautiful and famous. With all that she had going for her, why would she kill herself?

We cannot examine her life and thought processes the way we would our own. With a background of serious mental illness on her mother's side, an unstable upbringing, and a rather volatile history on her own part, her life certainly appears less glamorous in retrospect. She was treated for depression by a series of psychologists and psychiatrists and made several attempts at suicides. We cannot enter her cerebral cortex from her point of view and from a psychological standpoint give a definite yes or no to suicide. We can follow indications of what her actions and psychological makeup might have led to.

We can, nevertheless, analyze her life and hold it side by side with the scientific facts left by death. It is easy to want someone with such a remarkable life to have a sensational death. But sometimes the lives that fascinate us the most are not ones to be envied after all. And here, after a brief examination of the woman in life and a more thorough examination of the body in death, I must conclude that I agree with Dr. Tom Noguchi and with the 1982 investigation by the Los Angeles district attorney's office. I see no "credible evidence to support a murder theory."

Marilyn Monroe was beautiful and sought after, but she was also lonely and unhappy, and her tortured mind couldn't take it anymore. So with the pills that helped her make it through the night, she took her life.

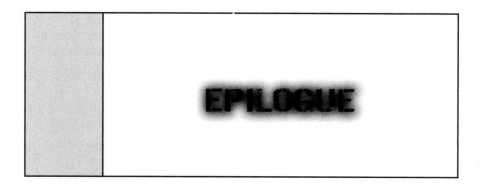

EPILOGUE

As the chapters in this book show, there are almost always different opinions about the same set of facts and circumstances in a given forensic case scenario. A frequently asked question is, how can that be—does not physical and biological evidence speak for itself, in a clear and unequivocal manner? The answer given by many individuals unfamiliar with the adversarial nature of the civil and criminal justice systems in the United States, or who simply distrust attorneys and are skeptical about all court-related endeavors, is that there exist a small percentage of dishonest, unscrupulous trial lawyers who will find unethical medical and scientific experts who are willing to prostitute themselves and provide whatever opinions are required for the right fee. While this kind of regrettable unprofessional conduct undoubtedly occurs, it does not fully and adequately explain why in nearly every high-profile case that proceeds to trial (and even those that never make it to the courtroom) top-flight experts with similar professional credentials and experience express antithetical conclusions about such seemingly basic and indisputable issues as cause, time, and place of death. (It is much more understandable that the manner of death, that is, natural, accident, suicide, or homicide, is likely to be contested in personal injury, workers' compensation, and homicide cases. Such differences of opinion will be encountered among forensic pathologists even in the absence of any known legal implications.)

What, then, is the most plausible explanation for these universally predictable adversarial confrontations? It is really rather simple. Medicine, including pathology (unquestionably the most concrete and tangible of all medical specialties), is not an absolute science. There is a significant component of subjective interpretation interwoven into the diagnostic process, understandably much more so in clinical situations. However, even after a complete autopsy with subsequent microscopic examination of tissues and toxicological analyses of body fluids, the specific cause of death may be in doubt. And, in many more cases, the manner of death will remain an arguable issue. That is why determination of time of death, exact location and position of the body when initially found, identification, correlation of preexisting natural disease processes or other injuries to the final mechanism of death, and sequence of deaths when more than one victim is involved are extremely important and relevant.

To complicate matters further, the sad and harsh, but undeniably true, fact is that a significant percentage of medicolegal postmortem examinations in the United States are still not being performed by formally trained forensic pathologists. Even more unfortunate is that some medical examiners and coroners, knowingly or subconsciously, develop a prosecutorial-related bias in criminal cases and a physician-protective bias in potential medical malpractice cases. As a result of these two highly relevant and severely compromising substantive and procedural negative factors, it is understandable that significantly different opinions will be encountered in many cases. Indeed, if every homicide case were to be handled by experienced, diligent attorneys, and if their clients had the financial wherewithal to retain appropriate consultants to review and evaluate the findings, conclusions, and opinions of the state's experts, the percentage of contested trials would be increased dramatically.

On a more benign basis, there is another interesting observation to make vis-à-vis forensic scientific investigations. Sometimes initial interpretations and seemingly obvious scenarios prove to be quite invalid upon further reflection. The statistical and experiential fact that certain things almost always happen in a well-known fashion does not necessarily mean that quite infrequently, or even very rarely, some other explanation of a most atypical, bizarre nature may not have been at play. This is an important concept that top-notch, objective, and truly independent forensic pathologists and other forensic scientists always keep in mind.

There can be a fine line of demarcation in many medicolegal deaths between the labeling of a case as an accident or a homicide, or sometimes as a suicide or even a natural death. Contrary to what is glamorously and fascinatingly depicted in popular television shows and best-seller novels, unequivocal and definitive biological, physical, or forensic evidence is not always to be found, despite the most scrupulous search. Nothing epitomizes that caveat more than the Peterson case.

The Scott Peterson case illustrates something that many people do not understand, namely, that someone can be convicted of first-degree murder based upon circumstantial evidence alone. It will be interesting to follow this case in future years to see if there is a successful appeal and a new trial.

The John F. Kennedy assassination investigation tragedy demonstrates incompetence at every turn. The fact that it occurred to such a monumental degree in the case of a president is truly astounding.

The Digman case is an example of how investigators can misinterpret the true nature of a case as a result of the failure to recognize and appreciate important physical features at the death scene.

Fame and fortune sometimes may result in a manipulation of the justice system. But on occasion, as the Jayson Williams case demonstrates, such individuals can be juicy targets for overly zealous prosecutors.

The public's infatuation with a beautiful celebrity like Marilyn Monroe will never permit her untimely death to be put to rest. Scientific reasoning and analysis, unfortunately, go out the window in a case like that. Suspicions of foul play can have a logical premise and should be thoroughly scrutinized and considered at the outset in analyzing such a case. But it is very difficult to disabuse legions of camp followers of their sinister interpretations once rumors concerning a popular performer's death have been disseminated.

The vagaries of clinical medicine and the unpredictability of death make it impossible to always explain the etiology of every patient's demise. The case of Jane Bolding serves to remind us that a provable charge of murder cannot be sustained by epidemiological data alone. Death doesn't always occur according to the numbers.

When the federal authorities decide to cover something up, they may well succeed. If they control the investigation and have a strong motivation to keep the truth from emerging, as in the Gander air crash, it is essentially impossible to crack the case open.

Police brutality in all instances, but especially when precipitated by racial bias, is unforgivable. The Gammage case is a glaring example of how an innocent person can be killed by out-of-control law enforcement tactics that need to be exposed by independent experts.

And then, of course, there is the very infrequent case in which no answer is forthcoming, despite thorough police investigation and analyses by expert forensic scientists. This is dramatically demonstrated by the Chandra Levy case. The manner of death can be reasonably conjectured, but the cause and time of death may be impossible to ascertain without other evidence forthcoming.

The authors earnestly hope that the readers of *Tales from the Morgue* will have found these true stories engrossing. And perhaps, more important, that you will have learned how good forensic science can contribute to a more effective, fair, and unbiased criminal justice system. A great democracy like ours cannot continue to thrive without such a commitment to the truth.

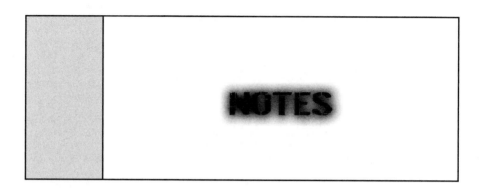

NOTES

Chapter 1. The Murder Trial of Scott Peterson: Sex, Lies, and Audiotape

1. "The Search for Laci Peterson—Chronology," *Modesto Bee*, April 22, 2003.

2. Harriet Ryan, "Peterson Researched Extensively before Bay Trip," Court TV, August 8, 2004.

3. Garth Stapley, "Police Talk to 4 Women," *Modesto Bee*, June 26, 2003.

4. Garth Stapley, "Peterson's House Sanitzed," *Modesto Bee*, September 20, 2004.

5. John Cote and Garth Stapley, "Scott Told Police There Were No Problems with Marriage," *Modesto Bee*, June 22, 2004.

6. Harriet Ryan, "Peterson Promptly Mentioned Suspect," Court TV, September 20, 2004, http://courttvcom/trials/peterson.

7. Brian Skoloff, "Detective Quickly Formed Theory," Associated Press, September 20, 2004.

8. Harriet Ryan, "Peterson Looks Away," Court TV, July 6, 2004.

9. Stapley, "Peterson's House Sanitized."

10. Ibid.

11. *Larry King Live*, CNN, January 13, 2003.

12. "Search for Laci Peterson," *ModestoBee.com*, April 22, 2003.

13. Ibid.

14. Associated Press, "Peterson Offered a Plea," August 6, 2003; Motion to Exclude Evidence filed by Mark Geragos.

15. "Search for Laci Peterson."

16. Ryan, "Peterson Looks Away."

17. Live Press Conference, NBC News, April 18, 2003; "Slam Dunk Remarks Live On," *Contra Costa Times*, April 19, 2003.

18. Contra Costa Coroner, Report of Autopsy 2003-0808.

19. John Cote, "Experts Examine Remains," *Modesto Bee*, August 12, 2003.

20. "Jury Seated in Peterson Trial," Associated Press, May 27, 2004.

21. Harriet Ryan, "Peterson Prosecutor Points to Loan of Circumstance Evidence," Court TV, June 1, 2004.

22. Harriet Ryan, "Two-Timer, Yes, but No Double Murderer," Court TV, June 2, 2004.

23. Ibid.

24. Brian Skoloff, "Laci's Stepfather Questioned on Fishing," Associated Press, June 9, 2004.

25. Harriet Ryan, "Expert Connects Peterson's Fishing Route to Location of Unborn Son," Court TV, October 4, 2004.

26. Harriet Ryan, "Tears, Tissues Injury Box," Court TV, September 16, 2004.

27. Harriet Ryan, "Peterson's Mistress Testifies," Court TV, August 10, 2004.

28. Ibid.

29. John Cote and Garth Stapley, "Frey Describes Romance," *Modesto Bee*, August 11, 2004.

30. "Peterson Found Guilty," *USA Today*, November 12, 2004.

31. Brian Skoloff, "Peterson Defense Offers Explanations," Associated Press, September 27, 2004.

32. John Cote and Garth Stapley, "Defense Tries to Paint Picture of Bias," *Modesto Bee*, September 29, 2004.

33. Garth Stapley and John Cote, "Peterson's Parents Get Chance to Testify," *Modesto Bee*, October 27, 2004.

34. Greta Van Susteren, *On the Record*, Fox News, October 27, 2004.

35. "Peterson Found Guilty."

36. Harriet Ryan, "Scott Peterson a Philanderer, Not a Killer," Court TV, November 11, 2004.

37. "Next Issue: Life or Death," *San Jose Mercury News*, November 27, 2004.

Chapter 2. Jayson Williams: One Last Game

1. *My Jayson Williams: Tanya Young Williams' Story*, http://myjayson williams.com/team/martin.html.

2. "Billy Martin's Opening Statement," *My Jayson Williams: Tanya Young Williams' Story*, http://myjaysonwilliams.com/documents/opening.html.

3. Jayson Williams with Steve Friedman, *Loose Balls* (New York: Doubleday, 2000), p. 240.

4. Harriet Ryan, "Gunshot Lands Williams in New Court," Court TV, January 13, 2004, http://courttv.com/trials/jaysonwilliams/background _ctv.html.

5. "Community Champions—Charitable Athletes," *Sporting News*, August 2, 1999, http://www.findarticles.com/p/articles/mi_m1208/is_31_223/ ai_55410353.

6. "Jayson Williams Gunplay Case, Witnesses for the Prosecution," CourtTV.com, http://www.courttv.com/trials/jaysonwilliams/witnesses _sta.html.

7. "Jayson Dodges Bullet," *New York Daily News*, May 1, 2004.

8. Adrian Wojnarowski, "Williams Had Too Much Time on His Hands," ESPN.com, February 28, 2002, http://sports.espn.go.com/nba /columns/story?columnist=wojnarowski _adrian&id=1342798.

9. Ibid.

10. David Aldridge, "The Rise and Fall of Jayson Williams," ESPN.com, http://sports.espn.go.com/nba/columns/story?columnist=aldridge_david&id =1342769.

11. Williams, *Loose Balls*, p. 232.

12. Ibid., p. 7.

13. Ibid., p. 122.

14. Harriet Ryan, "Damning Testimony against Williams, the 'Never

Mind,'" Court TV, February 19, 2004, http://www.courttv.com/trials /jaysonwilliams/021904_ctv.html.

15. Ibid.

16. "Jayson Williams Case Events List," My Jayson Williams: Tanya Young Williams' Story," http://myjaysonwilliams.com/trial/trial.html.

17. Ibid.

18. Associated Press, March 24, 2004.

19. Harriet Ryan, "Ex-teammate Certain Williams Pulled the Trigger," Court TV, March 4, 2004, http://courttv.com/trials/jayson williams/030404_ctv.html.

20. Ibid.

21. Robert Hanley, "Williams Trial Is Delayed over Dispute on Evidence," New York Times, April 6, 2004.

22. Giovanna Fabiano, "Judge Orders Williams Retrial Put on Hold," Bridgewater Courier News, February 18, 2005, http://www.c-n.com /apps/pbcs.dll/article?AID=/20050218/NEWS/502180326.

Chapter 3. Chandra Levy: Lost and Found

1. Chandra Levy timeline, "Washington Intern Missing More Than a Year, Found Dead," May 11, 2001, ABCNews.com.

2. Chandra Levy timeline, "Washington Intern Missing More Than a Year, Found Dead," Mid-January 2001, ABCNews.com.

3. Chandra Levy timeline, "Washington Intern Missing More Than a Year, Found Dead," May 7, 2001, ABCNews.com.

4. Key dates and events in Chandra Levy case, late May, Richard Willing, Donna Leinwand, and Kevin Johnson, "Levy Discovery Won't End Mystery," USA Today, May 23, 2002, p. 3A.

5. Chandra Levy timeline, "Washington Intern Missing More Than a Year, Found Dead," June 13, 2001, ABCNews.com.

6. Associated Press, "Police Still Haven't Determined Where Intern Died," New York Times, May 25, 2002, p. A14.

7. Mark Sherman, "Jury Hears from Condit Aide," Pittsburgh Tribune-Review, June 13, 2002, p. A18.

8. Mark Sherman, "Questions Still Surround Levy Mystery," Pittsburgh Tribune-Review, May 27, 2002, p. A4.

Chapter 4. The Case of Jonny Gammage: Death in Police Custody

1. Jim McKinnon, "Mystery Still Shrouds Fatal Arrest by Police," *Pittsburgh Post-Gazette*, October 18, 1995.

2. Ibid.

3. Jan Ackerman and Michael Fuoco, "Conflicting Accounts," *Pittsburgh Post-Gazette*, November 3, 1995.

4. Jim McKinnon and Johnna Pro, "Man Dies after Scuffle with Police," *Pittsburgh Post-Gazette*, October 13, 1995.

5. Ibid.

6. Ibid.

7. Johnna Pro, "Jackson Takes Up Gammage Death," *Pittsburgh Post-Gazette*, October 20, 1995.

8. Alan Robinson, "Seals' Cousin Died of Injuries in Police Custody," Associated Press, October 17, 1995.

9. McKinnon, "Mystery Still Shrouds Fatal Arrest by Police."

10. Mary Anne Lewis, "FBI to Study Seals' Cousin's Death," *Pittsburgh Tribune-Review*, October 18, 1995.

11. Michael A. Fuoco, Johnna Pro, and Ed Bouchette, "Neck, Chest Injuries Killed Motorist," *Pittsburgh Post-Gazette*, October 17, 1995.

12. Jim McKinnon, "Amid Rites, Syracuse Residents Deplore Loss of Gammage," *Pittsburgh Post-Gazette*, October 19, 1995.

13. Ibid.

14. Pro, "Jackson Takes Up Gammage Death."

15. Associated Press, "Five Police Officers Facing Charges in Beating Death," November 5, 1995.

16. Michael Fuoco, "Gammage Jury Asks Five Homicide Charges," *Pittsburgh Post-Gazette*, November 4, 1995.

Chapter 5. The Captain's Death: Suicide, Murder, or Accident?

1. "Case History," a thirty-page document prepared by Donna Digman on March 28, 1989.

2. Ibid.

3. Ibid.

4. Ibid.

5. Ibid.

6. Riverside County Sheriffs Office Investigative Report, January 22, 1989.

7. David Zucchino, "Marine's Parents Fight to Remove the Stain of Suicide," *Philadelphia Inquirer*, December 19, 1993.

8. Ibid.

9. "Case History."

10. Ibid.

11. Coauthor Mark Curriden interviewed Dr. Wecht and the Digmans extensively in recollecting their conversations on September 9, 2003.

12. Zucchino, "Marine's Parents Fight to Remove the Stain of Suicide."

13. Ibid.

14. Curriden interview with Dr. Wecht and the Digmans.

Chapter 6. Gander Air Crash: Ice or Sabotage?

1. Terri Taylor, "Gander Crash," *Investigative Reports*, Arts & Entertainment Network, March 20, 1992.

2. Ibid.

3. Ibid.

4. Canadian Aviation Safety Board (CASB), "Aviation Occurrence Report," October 28, 1988.

5. Taylor, "Investigative Reports."

6. Ibid.

7. CASB, "Aviation Occurrence Report."

8. Ibid.

9. Ibid.

10. Canadian Aviation Safety Board, "Dissenting Opinion," November 14, 1988.

11. Ibid.

12. Holly Gatling, "Four Years Later, Pieces in Crash Puzzle Still Don't Fit," *Columbia (SC) State*, December 11, 1989.

13. Ibid.

14. Taylor, "Investigative Reports."

15. Ibid.

16. Ibid.

17. Ibid.

18. Terri Taylor, *KDKA Evening News*, June 8, 1990.

19. Ibid.

20. Gatling, "Four Years Later, Pieces in Crash Puzzle Still Don't Fit."

21. Ibid.

22. Janet Crawley, "Did Icing Cause Crash of Arrow Air Flight," *Chicago Tribune Sunday Magazine*, April 22, 1990.

23. Ibid.

24. Ibid.

Chapter 7. Jane Bolding: Angel of Death or Victim of Statistics?

1. Julie Bell, "Making a Case in Patient Death May Be Difficult," *Baltimore Sun*, July 24, 2003.

2. Keith Harriston, "The Long, Tangled Path to a Nurse's Trial," *Washington Post*, May 15, 1988.

3. Ibid.

4. Ibid.

5. Ibid.

6. Ibid.

7. Keith Harrison, "Defendant as Victim," *Washington Post*, June 23, 1988.

8. Verbatim transcripts, Motion to Exclude Testimony, *State of Maryland v. Jane Bolding*.

9. Ibid.

10. *Miranda v. Arizona*, 384 U.S. 436 (1966).

11. Bell, "Making a Case in Patient Death May Be Difficult."

12. Centers for Disease Control, "Cluster of Unexplained Deaths at a Hospital," July 14, 1986.

13. Ibid.

14. Ibid.

15. Keith Girard, "Coffee Break with Lawyer Who Got Nurse Bolding Off the Hook," *Business Journal of Washington*, October 1988.

16. April Witt, "No Rest for the Suspects," *Washington Post*, June 4, 2001.

17. Keith Harriston, "Nurse Called Killer Angel," *Washington Post*, May 19, 1988.

18. Ibid.

19. Keith Harriston, "Bolding Predicted Patient's Death," *Washington Post*, May 27, 1988.

20. Ibid.

21. Keith Harriston, "Testimony Restricted in Nurse's Trial," *Washington Post*, June 2, 1988.

22. Keith Harriston, "Expert Rules Out Chance," *Washington Post*, June 7, 1988.

23. Keith Harriston, "Bolding Attorney Urges Directed Acquittal," *Washington Post*, June 16, 1988.

24. Keith Harriston, "Judge Acquits Nurse Bolding," *Washington Post*, June 21, 1988.

Chapter 8. Coup d'État: The Assassination of President John F. Kennedy

1. "The Motorcade," CourtTV Crime Library, www.crimelibrary.com.

2. Ibid.

3. Ibid.

4. Ibid.

5. Sixth-Floor Museum at Dealey Plaza.

6. Ibid.

7. *Warren Commission Report* (Washington, DC: Government Printing Office, 1964), p. 36.

8. Charles Crenshaw, *JFK: Conspiracy of Silence* (New York: Signet, 1992), pp. 118–19.

9. Mike Feinsalber, "JFK Autopsy Files Are Incomplete," Associated Press, August 2, 1998.

10. *Warren Commission Hearings* (Washington, DC: Government Printing Office, 1964), 2: 382.

11. *Warren Commission Report*, p. 580.

12. Verbatim transcript of press briefing from LBJ Library.

13. *Warren Commission Report*, p. 108.

14. Assassination Records and Review Board Medical Documents #44 and #86.

15. *Warren Commission Report*, p. 543.

16. Fred Graham, "Mystery Cloaks Fate of Brain of Kennedy," *New York Times*, August 27, 1972, p. 1.

17. Associated Press, "Expert: Rockefeller Commissioner Distorts View," June 11, 1975.

18. Letter of transmittal dated February 17, 1998, to Cyril Wecht from T. Jeremy Gunn, counsel to Assassinations Records Review Board.

19. *The Final Assassinations Report—Report of the Select Committee on Assassinations, U.S. House of Representatives* (New York: Bantam Books, 1979), p. 150.

20. Transcript of interview with Dan Rather provided to Cyril Wecht.

21. Memo by Richard Sprague, Chief Counsel, House Select Committee on Assassinations, record number 180-10086-10295.

22. "Testimony of Dallas Officer Bobby Hargis," *Warren Commission Report*, vol. 6, p. 294.

23. Dennis Breo, "JFK's Death," *Journal of American Medical Association*, May 27, 1992.

24. Assassinations Records and Review Board, Deposition of Floyd Albert Riebe.

25. George Lardner, "Archive Photos Not of JFK's Brain," *Washington Post*, November 10, 1998, p. A-3.

26. Ibid.

27. Warren Commission, Exhibit 1974, p. 25.

Chapter 9. "Good-Bye, Norma Jeane": The Death of Marilyn Monroe

1. Thomas T. Noguchi, MD, with Joseph DiMona, *Coroner* (New York: Simon & Schuster, 1983), p. 68.

2. Ibid., p. 56.

3. Ibid., p. 85.

4. "Mini-Biography of Marilyn Monroe," Court TV's Crime Library, http://www.crimelibrary.com/notorious_murders/celebrity/marilyn_monroe/2.html?sect=26.

5. Ibid.

6. "Danamo's Marilyn Monroe Online: Biography," http://marilynmonroepages.com/.

7. "Mini-Biography of Marilyn Monroe."

8. Diana Karanikas, *Marilyn: A Life in Pictures* (New York: Metro Books, 1999), p. 16.

9. Clark Kidder and Madison Daniels, *Marilyn Monroe unCovers* (Edmonton, AB: Quon Editions, 1994), http://glamournet.com/legends/Marilyn/.

10. Marilyn Monroe's Official Web site, biography, http://www.marilynmonroe.com/about/bio2.html.

11. Jim Dougherty, as told to L. C. Van Davage, *To Norma Jeane with Love* (Chesterfield, MO: BeachHouse Books, 2001).

12. "Danamo's Marilyn Monroe Online: Quotes," http://marilynmonroepages.com/.

13. Arthur Miller, *Timebends* (New York: Grove Press, 1987), p. 425.

14. "Remembering Marilyn Monroe," *Larry King Live*, June 1, 2001, http://transcripts.cnn.com/TRANSCRIPTS/0106/01/lkl.00.html.

15. "Candle in the Wind," music by Elton John, lyrics by Bernie Taupin, *Goodbye Yellow Brick Road*, MCA Records, 1973.

16. http://www.usps.com/images/stamps/95/marilyn.gif.

17. Page 2 Staff, "Let the Skirts Fly—Anna vs. Marilyn," ESPN.com, http://espn.go.com/page2/s/020404/annamarilyn.html.

18. Noguchi and DiMona, *Coroner*, p. 81.

19. Ibid.

20. Ibid.

21. Ibid., p. 77.

22. Ibid., pp. 78–80.

23. Ibid., p. 82.

24. Mailer, *Marilyn: A Biography*.

25. Cyril Wecht, Mark Curriden, and Benjamin Wecht, *Cause of Death* (New York: Onyx Books, 1993), p. 142.

26. "Limbaugh Admits Addiction to Pain Medication," CNN.com, October 10, 2003, http://www.cnn.com/2003/SHOWBIZ/10/10/rush.limbaugh/.

27. "Danamo's Marilyn Monroe Online: Quotes."

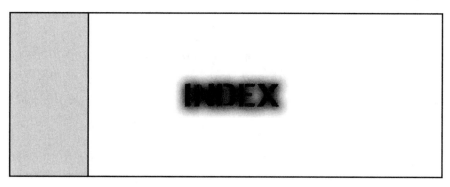

INDEX

PALISADES PARK PUBLIC LIBRARY, NJ

3 9153 09041297 6

Wecht, Cyril H.,
Tales from the morgue :forensic answers
Prometheus Books,2005.
39153090412976
Palisades Park Library

614.1
WEC